You Car ~

Sleep hygiene, hot baths, k
acupuncture, counselling, sup|

Over twenty years, I tried it al.. ..ouning worked. The more I tried to force sleep, the more I fed my anxiety and obsession – and the more insomnia stripped from my life.

I can't get up early as I can't sleep at night. I can't see my friends tonight. I can't do the job I love. I can't share a bed with my wife. I can't, I can't, I can't. For two decades, slowly but surely, insomnia took over my life and stole my happiness.

And then I found CBT-I. Everything changed. Every thought, every action, CBT-I had seen it all before. My insomnia was not unique. Your insomnia is not unique. It always boils down to two problems: sleep drive and hyperarousal.

By addressing both through behaviour changes, sleep knowledge and cognitive restructuring, I went from being somebody trying everything they could to make themself sleep to being somebody trying everything they could to stay awake.

After overcoming my insomnia, I trained with sleep physician Daniel Erichsen to help you overcome yours. In this book, I take you on my journey and share the gold-standard, evidence-based treatment so that *You Can Sleep Too!*

Joseph Pannell lives in sunny Devon where he surfs and walks his brown Dalmatian on the beach every day. Millions of people have insomnia, and he is a man on a mission to help every single one!

You Can Sleep Too!

Joseph Pannell

First published 2021

Cover design by Ross Embleton, an artist and designer based in North Devon who specialises in pencil drawings and logo design. If you would like something designed, you are welcome to email him at rossembleton@icloud.com.

TABLE OF CONTENTS

1

You Can Sleep Too!

People who have never had insomnia think you must be sleepy all the time. But that isn't it. You feel anxious, stressed, fatigued. A nervous, static, scratching gnawing energy like you would get from twenty espressos, but you never feel sleepy, ever. If you could somehow feel sleepy again, you would sleep...

My first episode of insomnia.

'Army, Navy or RAF?'

'Excuse me?' I said. A dark-haired woman, in her late fifties stood opposite me, pale skin, black eyes like two crows smashed into a chalk cliff. She repeated herself but louder and more insistently this time,

'Army, Navy or RAF?'

'Army,' I replied rather uncertainly. 'You should already have your boots, go down the corridor and pick up the remainder of your uniform from the second door on the left.' She then abruptly turned on her heel, and that was it, she was gone.

Within 30 minutes, I was on parade, having my brand-new boots inspected. Twenty minutes later, I was stripping down, cleaning, oiling and reassembling my L98A2 GP rifle. And 10 minutes after that, I was lying face down in the mud, loading live ammunition into a magazine, one eye closed looking down the sight at the black outline of my target. I heard a deep raspy voice and felt hot breath on my ear,

'Diaphragmatic breathing, remember, Joseph, long and slow, gently squeeze the trigger on the exhale.'

Shaking and sweating, my index finger gradually pulled backwards, a loud piercing crack and yes, yes, I had hit him, right in the centre of the chest. I heard a grunt of approval and felt his presence move away from me. It was then that I looked around me at my unit; like me they were all lying prostrate in the mud, dressed in identical camo, green and black painted faces, one eye staring fixedly down the barrels of their rifles. I was 14, Year 9, and on the second day at my new private school in Devon. At my old state school in Essex, we used to play dodgeball for PE. 'Where the hell am I?' I thought.

It was at my new school that I first suffered from my first bout of insomnia, something – though I didn't know it at the time – that would plague me for the next twenty years of my life. Nor did I know how easy it would have been to prevent, had I only known just three simple facts that I know today.

The school I had just left was your typical state secondary school with large, rectangular industrial buildings, chain-linked fences, run-down football pitches and a dreadful canteen that served chips and brown meat-like substances on plastic trays.

I had attended schools like this one my entire life. I understood the rules here. It was the 90s, so to fit in and be liked all you had to do was get yourself a bomber jacket and become either passable at football or be the one who always remembers to bring the ball. Simple!

My new school in Devon wasn't like this. It was a great, imposing Victorian building complete with stained-glass windows, turrets and buttresses.

Here, you ate three-course, well-balanced, organic meals at lunchtime. You did prep rather than homework, played rugby at breaktime, and on Tuesday evenings you sailed boats, flew aeroplanes or shot things. At my old school, I understood the rules and parameters. Marooned in a castle on the edge of a moor, I understood nothing.

There was also a barbarism to the place I had never encountered anywhere before.

After only two weeks of being there, I learnt how one of the boarders had been expelled for assaulting another with a soda bottle (he didn't hit him with it).

And after only two months, I myself was lured towards the squash courts and abruptly pushed inside, where I was confronted by my two opponents. Neither of them had a racket or a ball, but one of them did have a bicycle chain.

I heard a roar of cheers from the viewing gallery above and, looking up, saw a wall of jeering faces. It was only then I properly twigged what was happening, but it wasn't until the assembly the following day that I learnt the true scale of the event and the organisation behind it: multiple gladiatorial matches (some voluntary, some involuntary) in multiple squash courts, spanning all the year groups, complete with advertising posters and ticket sellers on the door.

I didn't come out of my conflict well, but perhaps better than expected, so I was left alone after that. But still, I wasn't precisely popular, so I just went into my shell. I think everyone assumed I was stupid because of it. I wasn't. I was just trying to stay out of people's way.

I was about four months into my two-year stretch at my new school when I first suffered from my first bout of insomnia.

I remember the first night it struck. It was the night after a geography lesson.

My Geography teacher was called Mr Steel. He wore suits that were always old and weather-beaten but expensive. He had a brown airstrip of hair, cheeks like underdone beef and liked to explain the four main types of coastal erosion in the most violent way possible.

'If I were to strap Ross to a cliff and the power of the waves were to smash against his face, and the air get trapped between his teeth and behind his eye sockets until they all fly out, leaving him a broken, mangled, bloody pulp, is that an example of attrition or hydraulic action, class?' (It's hydraulic action; his methods were extreme, but twenty years later I still remember, so they were effective.)

During that particular lesson, he had asked me to locate the Mediterranean on the map. I knew where it was, of course, I knew, but when he asked me, standing so uncomfortably close to me, he would paralyse me with fear to such an extent I could barely remember my name, much to the amusement and ridicule of the class.

Until that day, sleep had never been an issue; it had never been something I gave a second thought. I went to bed, I put my head on the pillow, and I would wake up. On the rare occasions when I was not in bed asleep, it didn't bother me. Quite the contrary, I was happy to be there, tucked up under the sheets all warm and cosy. I would sleep on my side, and I remember being so relaxed in bed that it was too much of an effort even to roll over. I took it for granted sleep would come, and it always did.

But that night was different. I lay in bed, and my mind replayed the thoughts from the day. Over and over, like a scratched record, distorted and echoing. And as I lay there, getting more and more anxious, new anxiety came over me. I realised I had been in bed for hours and that I wasn't asleep.

'How many hours exactly?' I thought. I pressed the light on my clock to look at the time. 12.32 am. I went to bed at 10.30, so I quickly did the maths. I had been awake for precisely 2 hours and 2 minutes. That only gave me a total of 5.28 minutes left in bed to sleep.

The old worry of the day was quickly replaced with the new fear that I would be tired the next day. What would happen to me if I wasn't able to function? I didn't want this to happen, so I tried to force sleep to come. And the more I forced, the more it evaded me, and the more anxious and stressed I got. I looked at the clock multiple times throughout the night. 1.42 am, 2.33 am, 3.44 am. When my alarm finally sounded, I felt like I had not slept at all.

Now you will understand better than anyone how a bad night's sleep makes you feel, so I am sure you will know that the next day I felt irritable, anxious and stressed. I spent the entire day wishing it would end so I could get back into bed, and as soon as I had the opportunity, I did just that. Despite not feeling sleepy, I went to bed far earlier than I would naturally go to bed to catch up on lost sleep. And for the second night in a row, I did not sleep.

As soon as I got into bed, I felt worried. Worried about the need to sleep and how I would feel the next day if I failed to sleep. Again, I lay there looking at the clock, counting the minutes until they slowly drained away until the morning. I felt sweaty and hot, and I felt angry with myself. I had put even more effort in this second night than the first because the need to sleep was even greater, but still, sleep didn't come.

But am I the only one who has ever done this? I'm going to break the fourth wall and speak directly to you. Does anything I have just written resonate with you? The trigger for your first sleepless night(s) will have been different from mine. And maybe your type of sleeplessness was different too. Perhaps you fell asleep without any trouble but woke up and couldn't get back to sleep. Or possibly you woke early in the morning and then remained awake. Or perhaps you had a whole night of poor, fragmented, broken sleep.

But are clock-watching and anxiety, trying to force sleep and anger when you fail, going to bed when you are not sleepy to catch up on sleep, and worry about what will happen to you if you don't sleep things you have experienced? Possibly you are already starting to see at least some similarities between my insomnia and your own. If that is the case, maybe your own, very different, special, personal insomnia isn't entirely unique after all. Very good!

As this may be the case, the evidence-based Sleep Knowledge snippets that I dot throughout the book will therefore be as astoundingly helpful to you as they were to me. I learnt them during my own sleep course and met them again subsequently when I was studying to become a sleep coach with sleep physician Daniel Erichsen and when exploring the resources and scientific studies freely available from the Sleep Medicine programmes run by Harvard and Oxford University.

And the first Sleep Knowledge section is coming up, now!

Sleep Knowledge 1
It does not matter what first triggered your insomnia

What first triggered your insomnia may be something as seemingly trivial as my own experience, or it may be something incredibly distressing. However, the evidence shows that it is not what is causing your insomnia to continue.

Stressful and distressing events can and do cause short-term sleep problems, as do changes in medication, illnesses, aches and pains and a whole host of other circumstances that cannot possibly be avoided. Virtually every person on the planet will experience a short-term sleep problem at some point in their life, for one reason or another. But for the majority of people, this does not develop into long-term insomnia.

Suppose you were to take my case as an example. I had a hard time at school twenty years ago. However, I know loads of people who also had a hard time at school. They may have experienced a short-term sleep problem, but they did not develop insomnia. Certainly not for twenty years.

Perhaps your insomnia was triggered by an apparently insignificant event like mine, or perhaps the trigger was something much more traumatic. Perhaps it was some medication, or an ailment, or perhaps it was simply put down to ageing.

But do you know somebody, or know of somebody, who has experienced something similar, has the same ailment, is on the same medication, or is the same age who does not have insomnia?

I thought my insomnia was unique. It wasn't. Everybody I speak to thinks their insomnia is unique. It isn't. The things that cause a short-term sleep problem to become insomnia and to allow insomnia to continue are

1. behaviours
2. thought patterns which lead to hyperarousal.

That's it! Nothing else.

I will go into much greater detail about hyperarousal throughout the book, but for now, hyperarousal is any type of heightened alertness such as anger, stress, anxiety or **excitement**.

Hyperarousal is accompanied by a physiological change in the body – the increase of adrenaline, cortisol, heart rate and body temperature. It is the body's threat-response mechanism that makes you alert, to keep you safe!

But, Joseph, I am safe, and there is no threat. So what's hyperarousal got to do with my insomnia? Everything! And I'll get to why that is later on I promise.

So my behaviours and thought patterns were what caused me to develop insomnia over the long term. The trigger had nothing to do with it.

I have already started to lay out what a few of these behaviours and thought patterns were (forcing sleep is a big one), and I will go into them in more detail in the following chapters. When you read about them, you will inevitably see a few differences between your own insomnia behaviours and thought patterns and mine. But perhaps you will also see similarities. Even if they are only slight, keep an eye out for these similarities. They will be incredibly beneficial to you because they mean that the same thing that I used to escape my insomnia can also banish yours!

2

Perpetuating the Problem

I had slept poorly for four days in a row, but finally, the week-end rolled around. I had been looking forward to this more than usual. Not just so I could be away from school for a couple of days, but so I could also finally catch up on some sleep.

On Friday night, stressed and anxious about what the night would bring, I went to bed early in the hope of catching up on sleep.

I woke at midday relieved; my anxiety and stress lifted clean off of me. It had taken me hours of force, pleading, bargaining and negotiating, but around 4 am, I had been able to drop off.

By sleeping on into the afternoon after four long days of sleep-lessness, I had eventually managed what I had been after – 8 hours of deep, uninterrupted sleep. It took me 13 hours in bed to get it, but I had finally managed to achieve what I wanted.

I quickly did the maths. Had it had been a weekday when I had to get up at 7 am, I would have only slept for 3 hours. But by lying in bed until noon, I had managed eight! Precisely the amount of sleep I thought we all needed.

Surfing, skiing, language learning… As with virtually every-thing in life, the more time you spend doing something and the harder you try, the greater the likelihood that you will succeed. By sleeping late into the day and getting what I was after, I had just proved to myself that sleep was no different.

I was 14 years old when I first had this thought. But it was reward and repetition that turned this thought into the fixed belief that would turn a short-term sleep problem into the long-term chronic insomnia that I suffered with for twenty years.

For the next two months, weekends were my saviour. Despite going to bed early every night to give myself as much opportunity as possible, most nights I still couldn't achieve the full 8 hours that I had always been told (by television, media, common knowledge) I needed.

But the weekends were different. By sleeping late into the afternoon, I could always force myself to sleep at the weekends.

Most weekdays, however, were not like the weekends. Although occasionally, through strategy and ingenious techniques, they were. Before I had ever had a sleep problem, all I needed to do to sleep was to feel sleepiness come, go to bed, and I would sleep. This was no longer happening, so I came up with ever more elaborate and creative ways to make sleep happen.

I slept at the north end of the bed. One night that worked, so I slept at the north end of the bed every night. That stopped working, so I would alternate between north and south, and some nights I would sleep, and some nights I wouldn't. But it seemed to help sometimes. That was my reward. Sometimes I slept! I wanted to sleep and, through action, I had made myself sleep, so I stuck at it. Sticking at it was my repetition.

I tried two pillows instead of one. That worked. Until it stopped working. But it had worked before, so some nights I would try two pillows, and some nights I would try one. And some nights I would sleep at the north end of the bed with two pillows, and some nights I would sleep at the south end of the bed with one.

Before the internet there was Teletext. I had a tiny fat-backed telly at the end of my bed. One night, I found that if I looked at the Teletext picture and squinted my eyes until the image started to blur, I would fall asleep afterwards. It was a form of relaxation and meditation technique I had invented. Aren't I clever, I thought! And sometimes it worked, and sometimes it didn't.

Sometimes I slept at the south end of the bed with two pillows and watched Teletext. And sometimes I slept at the north end of the bed with one pillow and didn't watch Teletext. And sometimes I would listen to light music while watching Teletext at the north end of the bed with three pillows (two under my head, one under my feet) after doing a visualisation exercise but before doing a muscle relaxation exercise. But only if I had had a warm bath two hours before bed, or if it was a Tuesday and I had had two kiwi fruit (for the melatonin), a glass of hot milk, moved my dressing gown onto the lower peg and rubbed my boxer dog's belly for luck...

These were my weekday behaviours and rituals. In just a couple of months, I had already built up quite a large number, but these paled into insignificance compared to what I eventually managed over twenty years.

I thought these behaviours were helping me sleep. Now I know with absolute certainty these behaviours fed my insomnia.

Sleep Knowledge 2
Your behaviours and thought patterns perpetuate your insomnia

If you take a look at the behaviours that caused and perpetuated my insomnia, you can see I was

> ➤ going to bed when I was not can't-keep-my-eyes-open sleepy to try and force 8 hours' sleep;
> ➤ massively extending my time in bed and indulging in obsessive, ritualistic behaviours to force sleep;
> ➤ waking up late in the day to prioritise short-term sleep over long-term, good-quality, regulated sleep;
> ➤ napping during the day (actually, I hadn't started this habit yet, but this comes later!).

From the lofty position of hindsight, and only after completing a sleep course, I now see that none of my short-term strategies helped me sleep. However, what they did do was increase my anxiety and obsessive thoughts around sleep, turn my bed into a place of stress and worry, and give me more trouble sleeping by deregulating my sleep drive (I will discuss the sleep drive in far greater detail throughout the remainder of this book).

I was trying to help myself, but I ended up making things a lot worse. Why did I do this?

To answer this question, it is helpful to understand that the brain is hard-wired to monitor threats and to keep us safe; it's how we survive! Due to circumstances beyond my control, I had a lot of trouble sleeping. I – like everybody at some point in their life – had a short-term sleep problem.

If I had known what to do – just accepted this fact and done nothing – I wouldn't have developed insomnia. But I didn't do nothing. During a stressful event, poor sleep is normal, but at the time, my 'fight or flight' brain didn't see it this way. The amygdala, the part of the brain that keeps you out of harm's way, identified lack of sleep as a threat. It saw it as a threat that I had to fight. So I changed my behaviours: I got up late, I spent longer in bed, and because I didn't understand that the only thing that can produce sleep is wakefulness, I had more trouble sleeping.

The more trouble I had sleeping, the more I craved sleep. And the more I longed to sleep, the more anxious, worried and stressed about not sleeping I became. And the more anxious I became about not sleeping, the more trouble I had sleeping. And the more trouble I had sleeping, the more I adapted my behaviours to force sleep. And the more I adapted my behaviours to force sleep, the more trouble I had sleeping. And the more trouble I had sleeping, the more desire ... You can see where I'm going here!

By craving, worrying and obsessing about sleep, I was telling my brain there was a threat (though there wasn't; poor sleep from time to time is normal), and the brain responded by doing what it always does when there is a threat: it made me anxious, so I could respond to that threat!

How did I respond? I modified my behaviours. I wanted good-quality, regulated sleep. But were sleeping late, napping and spending hours and hours in bed the behaviours of somebody who wants good-quality regulated sleep? Definitely not! They were the behaviours of somebody who wanted fragmented, poor quality, unregulated sleep. That's what I asked for, and that's what my body gave me.

From what you have read so far, I bet you can think of a couple of ways that your insomnia is different from mine (perhaps you wake in the middle of the night and have trouble falling back to sleep or you wake very early in the morning). But I also bet there are more similarities between my insomnia and your insomnia than there are differences. I had insomnia, so I had two problems:

1) a sleep-drive problem (caused and perpetuated by my behaviours)
2) a hyperarousal problem (caused and perpetuated by my behaviours).

Perhaps if your insomnia is more similar to mine than it is different, possibly it isn't unique after all; maybe you have these two problems too. If that is the case, that's good news because I'll be discussing them both in a later Sleep Knowledge section of the book!

3

A Brief Break and My Second Episode

Aged 14, I had my first episode of insomnia, and it lasted for about two months. And then, as abruptly as it had started, it ended.

I went to bed on a weekday expecting the same battle for sleep, but, for some reason, that night the conflict never came. I went to bed, and I slept. I slept the same as I had always done. No rituals, no obsessive behaviours, I just went to bed, closed my eyes and woke up six and a half hours later.

The next night, even though I had slept well the night before, I again felt sleepy, and again I went to bed, closed my eyes and woke up six and a half hours or so later. No forcing. No fighting. Nothing.

This is strange, I thought. So I put my brain into action and searched for the meaning behind how and why this had happened. I said to myself:

'Well, the summer holidays are coming up soon, so I'm no longer stressed or anxious about school.'

and

'Things are going a little better lately. I did well in a test the other day.'

I took a bus ride through my brain, looking for meaning, and I concluded that when life is going well, I can sleep, and when it is going badly, I can't. I have an over-active mind I said to myself, so when things are difficult, I think more, but when things are easier, I don't have that, so –

That was the meaning I placed on my first episode of insomnia. This meaning wasn't based in reality. There had been difficult times previously in my life when I had been stressed or worried or unhappy, and sleep had always come. But people need certainty. I needed some way to try to explain my insomnia, somewhere to hang my hat, and this is the hook I found for it.

At age 14, I had my first episode of insomnia. After that, I slept well for two years, and the fear of not sleeping was not something that crossed my mind.

At 16, I had left my old private school for a state-run college which I loved; things were going wonderfully well. Although my first episode was a horrible time in my life, I had put it behind me, and I didn't worry about insomnia returning. But it did return, and the reason for it seems so trivial that I am almost embarrassed to mention it.

I was sick – sticky, amorphic mass clutching-the-porcelain sick. I had been splayed out on the toilet floor for hours. I should have stayed there, but I didn't. It was 8 am, and I had a job interview in an hour – weekend bakery assistant at a local supermarket. My friend already worked there, it paid over £4 an hour and, apparently, if you pretended to drop them, you could eat as many *pains au chocolat* as you liked.

This wasn't something I was going to miss, but in hindsight, it would have been wise. At 9 am, smelling like a ferret cage and with the ghostly, pimpled, dishevelled complexion of an underdone punched ham quiche, I found myself knocking on the black painted wooden door of an interview room.

'Come in!' said a bright female voice. As I entered, she greeted me. She was mid-twenties, chestnut hair, very beautiful and wearing a dress that for a job interview was cut on the borderline of social acceptability.

I remember this distinctly because when I stretched out my hand to shake hers, I projectile vomited right into it.

Those who have led colourful lives will probably see this as nothing more than some light shading. At worst, it could be seen as cringeworthy. At best, a clear demonstration of my commitment and desire for the position (I didn't get the job).

You might think that this – admittedly embarrassing –experience certainly shouldn't have been enough to trigger – let alone justify – eighteen years of insomnia. And you would be right to think that. And it wasn't. But my return to the behaviours and belief patterns I had learnt during my first episode of insomnia was.

I got back from my job interview and tucked myself into bed, determined to sleep. But, head spinning from the stress and embarrassment of it all, I didn't. The next night I didn't either. But the second night I wasn't anxious about what happened; I had more or less laughed that off.

What I was anxious about now was not sleeping. Even though I had had two years of sleeping well, my mind suddenly chose to laser in on my two-month episode of insomnia.

What you focus on you attract. Rather than focusing on the fact that I had proven to myself that I was a good sleeper, to keep me safe, my mind instead focused on my inability to sleep. As soon as my mind did this, the old thought patterns came back – the anger, the torment and the frustration. And washed in on the tide of my old thought patterns came the old behaviours and techniques to force sleep.

One pillow, two pillows, north end of the bed, south end of the bed, squinting at the telly, relaxation techniques … Just the same as before. And just the same as before, I went to bed when I wasn't sleepy to force 8 hours of sleep, lying in bed for hours not sleeping and becoming more and more angry and frustrated. Whenever possible, I would get up late in the day in order to catch up on sleep.

None of this had fixed my insomnia before, and none of this fixed my insomnia now. But desperate for sleep and in the absence of any knowledge that would help me sleep, I didn't know any better.

Sleep Knowledge 3
The 8 hours' sleep myth

Do you think you need 8 hours of sleep? Actually, people who sleep for 8 hours are not typical.

The average time spent in bed among people who do not have a sleep problem is closer to 7 hours, and the time actually spent asleep is a little over 6 hours.

Below is an excerpt from my sleep tutor Daniel Erichsen's book *Set It & Forget It*.

> Studies show that when healthy adults with no sleep problems are asked, their belief is that they get 7 hours of sleep.
>
> In reality, most people don't have a clue.
>
> Either they simply guess that they sleep about 7 hours because it sounds about right or they'll assume that they sleep 7 hours because they go to bed at 11 pm and get up at 6 am. When you objectively examine these same people, a different story emerges. Using electroencephalography (EEG) or actigraphy (think Fitbit) you find that their average sleep is actually a bit above 6 hours. Objectively measured, more adults sleep between 5.5 and 7 hours.
>
> In other words, people with no trouble sleeping overestimate how much they sleep by about 1 hour. When we

look at quality instead of quantity, things are very similar. Those without sleep problems believe they don't wake up during the night or only wake up a few times. In fact, when you study someone in a sleep lab, seeing a couple of awakenings **every hour** is the norm.

Again, most don't have a clue what is going on. They wake multiple times but fall back asleep quickly and don't remember all the times they were awake during the night. (Erichsen 2020, pp. 16–17)

When objectively measured, people with no sleep problems **overestimate** how much they sleep.

When objectively measured, people with insomnia **underestimate** how much they sleep.

Before my sleep course, I used to think that I needed 8 hours' sleep, and I would spend, 11, 12, 13 hours in bed trying to achieve this, getting more and more anxious when I wasn't able to.

After regulating my sleep during my course, I now know that 6.5 hours of good-quality, regulated sleep works perfectly for me.

But that is for me. And everybody is different. How much sleep you need will be different. The amount of sleep you personally need is just enough to feel refreshed the next day. That's it.

You probably don't know how much sleep you need yet, but you will. Perhaps you may need less than me. Maybe you need more. But comparing yourself to a long sleeper or aiming to sleep for 8 hours every night (which very few people do) only increases anxiety when you fall short of this and leads to you spending more time in bed awake and not sleeping.

And so you enter a vicious circle where you become agitated and stressed about not sleeping, making it even harder for sleep to come.

Perhaps you think that you need to spend more time in bed to encourage (or possibly force, persuade, beg!) sleep to come. I know from personal experience that the opposite is true. Deliberately limiting the length of time you spend in bed (sleep restriction) is one of the critical components of CBT-I. NATTO uses a variation on this technique – the sleep window. Sleep windows deliver not only incredibly rapid but astoundingly successful results. I will cover them in much greater detail later in the book.

I've just thrown a new acronym at you out of nowhere: NATTO – non-attachment to the outcome.

To overcome my own insomnia, I completed a CBT-I course, which was amazing, and I am incredibly thankful to have found it. I then took a NATTO course with Daniel Erichsen, so I could learn to become a sleep coach in order to help others sleep by writing this book. I don't think there is another course like it, so I was also extremely glad to have found that one too.

There are differences (for example, as explained above, CBT-I advocates sleep restriction while NATTO uses a sleep window) but also many similarities between the two approaches. Both courses were enormously helpful to me, so I have picked aspects from both of them to share with you.

I have included a link to Daniel Erichsen's YouTube channel in the resources section so that you can learn more about NATTO. When you do, you will notice how I use the philosophy of NATTO in this book.

So, while the NATTO philosophy informs the whole of this book, my sleep course was CBT-I, so that will be the course I am describing when I talk about the specifics of my course.

4

Insomnia and Relationships

Four years on from my unfortunate incident in the interview room, in the third year of university, at the age of 20, I had a little better luck with women and met my ex-wife. For the purposes of this book, I'm going to call her Claire.

Usually during books such as these, the narrative is that our eyes met across a crowded room, and I thought she was the most beautiful woman I have ever met. You know the rest. This wasn't the case for me. When our eyes first met, I thought she looked rank.

Before you get angry with me for saying so, I'm only doing it because it's wrong to lie, and it is the truth. It is the truth because it was Claire's intention.

Claire was dressed as a granny. I know most are gorgeous and glamorous, but she was deliberately not. Blue rinse in curlers, lipstick on the teeth, shapeless floral dress ten sizes too big, Zimmer frame, shopping bags, the whole works. She was also drunk off her box, and she and her gaggle of grannies wouldn't leave me alone. I bore the bruises from the walking sticks for three days as testament to the fact.

Frankly, I wasn't into her, but Aberystwyth being a small place meant that I bumped into her again. And when I did, I did indeed think she was beautiful. She had alive, smiling eyes that let me know I was in a whole world of trouble. We had the best time together.

I think we fell for each other because we excited each other; we pushed each other to do things outside our comfort zone. To make some extra money, Claire life modelled. So not to be outdone I did so too. Standing naked in front of a room full of people (mostly women) measuring you up by doing that thing where you place your thumb on a pencil is slightly disconcerting. Especially when you knew a fair few of them and would probably bump into them the following evening on a night out.

But she did it. So I did. For my part, I surfed and was a qualified skydiver. I have always had a morbid fascination with doing things that scare me. I don't even like heights. If there is a high bridge with a barrier, I struggle to look over the side, and on a hot air balloon trip I once strapped myself into the basket with my belt in case I fell out.

But despite this, I jumped because I had an attraction to adventure and doing the things that terrify me the most.

I have always been like this. In my formative years in playschool, I would continuously summit the climbing frame and launch myself off. I also used to escape through a hole in the fence to play in the woods. The day I was expelled, after an hour-long search, I was found wedged inside a badger set.

My sleep was poor at university but not as bad as it had been. Many of my seminars didn't start until late morning or early afternoon, and an irregular sleep pattern was in no way abnormal among my peers. This lack of structure and regularity cemented the habit of 'catching up' on sleep by waking up late in the afternoon.

When we left university, Claire and I ended up in Cornwall living in a static caravan at the back of a farm in Perranporth. Claire worked at a riding school down the road, and I at a little theme park called Miniatura Park (the world in miniature – lofty, awe-inspiring landmarks like the Statue of Liberty and the Eiffel Tower shrunk down until they became considerably less impressive. There were also plastic dinosaurs – but the park doesn't exist anymore.)

It was while living together in Cornwall that Claire learnt the full extent of my insomnia. Fun as our jobs were, they didn't precisely afford us a lavish lifestyle, so we each had a blow-up mattress as our bed.

I would always go to bed at the same time as her, which was nearly always around 10.30 pm, and Claire would more often than not rise at about 7 am. Claire was a rarity. Unlike the majority of the population, she did indeed sleep for roughly around 8 hours most nights. And thinking at the time that this was the norm, I tried to force 8 hours too.

When Claire got up at 7 am in the morning and, cup of tea in hand, opened the static caravan door to take in the morning sun, she would regularly find me in the field, next to the chicken shed, with an eye mask over my face.

Outdoor sleeping was another bizarre ritual I had adopted. The stress and anxiety of crunching in a ball, kicking out my legs, continually moving and rotating as I tried to grab hold of my greasy insomnia and wrestle it to submission caused all the nerve endings in my body to feel like it was on fire.

Feeling roasting hot isn't something unique to me; it was a physiological response. The cortisol and adrenaline coursing through me from the anxiety and stress were causing my heart rate and temperature to sky rocket. (Perhaps you feel hot at night too …)

To combat this, one night, I took my mattress outside where it was cooler. It worked, I slept! As with my other bizarre, obsessive behaviours and rituals, my brain linked me sleeping outside next to a chicken coop to the positive outcome I was after – sleep.

And, as before, sometimes sleeping outside worked, and sometimes it didn't. But there was another reason why I chose on occasion to sleep outside. It was easier this way. I wanted to sleep next to my partner, of course, I did, but I didn't want to suffer next to her. If I was going to suffer, it was easier to do it alone.

It was in Cornwall that I learnt how well my Claire slept. I secretly envied this. While I would never wish insomnia on anybody, especially someone that I loved, there was a part of me that wished everybody could experience it for just a short time. Not because I wanted them to have it, but only so I knew that they understood.

Friends, partners, family, even the doctor you go to see who you think would understand, you quickly find out, don't understand insomnia. And you can't help people to understand it either.

You can't help people understand insomnia because until you learn a way out of insomnia, you don't really understand it yourself. You don't know why you always wake up in the middle of the night at the same time and can't fall back to sleep. You don't understand why you find it easier to fall asleep late in the morning but can't fall asleep earlier on in the night or why you wake early every morning, why you have to have your bed in a certain way or have to perform a certain ritual.

You know the anxiety and how you feel about it, but you can't explain it. You're by yourself. Insomnia has a way of making you feel very lonely like that.

'The eye sees not itself But by reflection' is one of my favourite lines from Shakespeare and very apt in explaining why I found it easier not sleep next to my partner when my insomnia was at its worst.

You see, she was my mirror. She didn't sleep like a normal sleeper. (Did you know 'normal sleepers' only sleep well roughly 70% of the time, which means that it is prevalent for most people to sleep poorly approximately one night in three? Well, that's true and something I will go into in more detail later on.)

Although even she had the occasional poor night's sleep, the vast majority of nights she didn't.

Claire would glide virtually every night into a deep sleep – no fighting, no force; it was effortless for her. Every night she would be in a place I was desperate to get to but couldn't. The stark contrast between her and me was the mirror that reflected how abnormal I and my sleep were. 'There is something wrong with me', I would think.

Claire always seemed to sleep well as she seemed to possess something I didn't. My nickname for what **made** Claire sleep was 'the wall'. She would be carrying on as usual and then around about 10.30 at night it was like she had hit a brick wall. Her mind and body would shut down, and she just had to go to bed. I was different. I didn't have a wall, ever.

Sleep eventually came after hours of pleading, bargaining, grappling, fighting. Still, I never had that beautiful sleepy feeling where your eyelids start to feel heavy, and, like an old tapestry, your mind begins to fray at the edges as the threads unravel.

Sleep never picked me up abruptly and pitched me over the black mercurial edge.

But it used to, I remembered that it used to.

It turned out, however, that 'the wall' is called 'the sleep drive' and that I did still have one. I just needed to change my behaviours and know the right action to switch it back on.

Sleep Knowledge 4
The sleep drive and hyperarousal

Insomnia boils down to two problems: unregulated sleep drive and hyperarousal.

Sleep drive

Below is an excerpt from 'Healthy Sleep' by Harvard Medical School's Division of Sleep Medicine. I will be posting a link to the article on the resources page at the back of this book. The resources page will also contain links to sleep courses, books, apps and recommended YouTube videos. So wherever you are based in the world and whatever your budget, I've got you covered!

> Scientists refer to sleep drive as a homeostatic system. Like body temperature or blood sugar, sleep is regulated internally. For instance, when body temperature falls, blood vessels constrict and we shiver; when blood sugar levels rise, the pancreas secretes insulin; and

when we remain awake for an extended period of time, structures in the brain promote sleep.

Furthermore, the duration and depth of our sleep vary according to the quantity and quality of sleep obtained previously.

With every waking hour there is a strengthening of the homeostatic sleep drive. This strengthening isn't directly measurable as a quantity, but experts think that it is the result of the level of brain activity during wakefulness. One hypothesis suggests that the build-up in the brain of adenosine, a by-product of energy consumption by cells, promotes sleep drive. (Division of Sleep Medicine at Harvard Medical School 2007, n.p.)

Simply put, the longer you are awake, the stronger your sleep drive will become.

To provide a simple analogy to show how the sleep drive works, I present to you 'John'.

John's a normal sleeper and generally doesn't have trouble sleeping most nights. He sleeps for around 6.5 hours.

To generate 6.5 hours of sleep, he needs to have 17.5 hours of wakefulness.

He usually wakes at 6.30 am. So he will start to feel sleepy as it approaches midnight.

But if John wakes up at 9.30 am one day and needs 17.5 hours of wakefulness to feel sleepy, when will he feel sleepy the following day?

For those of you who failed GCSE maths, it's around 3 am.

'But', I hear you say 'I don't sleep. Most nights I only sleep for 4, 5, 6, hours, and some nights it feels like I get no sleep at all, but I still have no sleep drive.'

That's what I said! And those were my objections. But sleep deprivation and insomnia are not the same thing. (I will discuss this more in the next Sleep Knowledge section.)

Another reason that you may not feel sleepy, or you may not perceive sleepiness, is hyperarousal.

Hyperarousal

Is any type of heightened alertness such as anger, stress, anxiety or excitement. (As a child, did you ever feel so excited before Christmas Day you couldn't sleep? That was hyperarousal!)

Now I present to you 'Vicky'.

Vicky does not have a sleep problem either. For her holiday, she goes on a wild camping trip to a national park. After hiking deep into the woods, she pitches her tent just before nightfall and, tucked up in her sleeping bag at roughly 11 pm, starts to feel sleepy. Normally she would fall asleep no problem, but just as she is about to drift off, she hears the howl of a wolf that sounds much too close to her tent for comfort. Listening closer she hears the scratch, scratch, scratching of a tree and the bellowing of a grizzly bear.

What's the chance of Vicky falling asleep while all that is going on?

No chance whatsoever. She's going to be alert, anxious, stressed. Her heart rate, body temperature, adrenaline and cortisol will all increase, and she will be poised, ready for fight or flight.

She is not going to fall asleep because wolves and bears present a real tangible threat to Vicky's safety.

Not sleeping is not a tangible threat. You will not get gnashed by something with big spiky teeth if you are safely tucked up in a house and you do not sleep on a given night.

> But if you have insomnia and you fear not sleeping, then you have yourself a **perceived threat**, and the brain cannot tell the difference between a perceived threat and an actual threat.
>
> Every time you are fighting insomnia, worrying about not sleeping, getting angry with yourself, pleading with insomnia, counting down the minutes until the morning, you are telling your body that there is a threat to your safety, that there is a wolf in the bedroom and it better prep itself for fight or flight. And it does. It raises your heartbeat, blood pressure, body temperature, adrenaline and cortisol. This is called hyperarousal, and hyperarousal if strong enough can mask the sleep drive.

When it comes to whether or not you will sleep, it is simple.

1) No sleep drive + No hyperarousal = Relaxed and happy, but not asleep

2) No sleep drive + Hyperarousal = Feeling stressed and anxious, and not asleep

3) Sleep drive + Hyperarousal = You are sleepy, but your hyperarousal masks your sleep drive, and you are not asleep

4) Sleep drive + No hyperarousal = Sleep!

That's sleep in a nutshell. If you have a drive to sleep and you are not hyperaroused, you will sleep.

5

Skiing and Napping

After our time in Cornwall, Claire and I lived in a ski resort in the French Alps called Les Arcs. Here we ran a chalet, and I ski guided. It was a fantastic experience. We would cook breakfast for the guests in the morning, clean the chalet and, before the baking of the afternoon tea and evening dinner, we would hit the slopes.

But there was a problem. I had to get up at 6 am every morning for breakfast prep. Knowing this before bed every night caused my anxiety to surge, and I would spend the whole night wrestling with sleep.

Some nights it came, eventually, but when it didn't, which I felt was frequently, I would catch up on sleep after we had finished breakfast with an extended nap at 11o'clock.

I hadn't been able to nap before, but now in France having to get up at 6 am, I would sleep immediately every morning at 11 am. Always.

At night I had the usual battle for sleep, but at 11 am I could sleep fine, so I would sleep for 1.5 to 2 hours.

Me napping caused a massive crack in our relationship. Claire wanted to ski with me. Of course she did, that's what we had come to France to do. And I wanted to ski too; I love it, I always have. All of it, planning the day's route, sitting on a chairlift with a hot chocolate, exploring little offshoots between the trees, watching the bored and mildly cross French ski instructors and the snake of little bundled up 5-year-old starfishes crash into the back of each other behind them. It's wonderful! Every second of it.

But I needed sleep. I was desperate to feel human again, and if I just took those 2 hours, I could enjoy the rest of the day. It wasn't ideal, I thought, but it's better.

'But I don't understand it,' she would say, 'Why can you sleep now but not at night? It doesn't make any sense.' She was angry. I felt selfish, but I needed sleep, and that's the way I had learnt to get it. And I didn't understand it either, but I do now.

Like food and like water, my body needed sleep. It had a strong drive for it and by forcing it to get 8 hours at night, spending most of it battling and not getting good-quality sleep, it had adapted; I had conditioned it to give me sleep at 11 am.

The pressure was also off at 11 am. As well as a strong drive to sleep, I also believed that I could sleep at 11 am. Not at night-time. No. I believed I couldn't sleep at night-time, so when I went to bed, I was hyperaroused. But 11 am was different. I can always sleep at 11 am I told myself. I had complete confidence in my ability to sleep at 11 am, so I wasn't hyperaroused and had a strong drive to sleep. So I slept.

Back then, I set my sleep time to 11 am. Now that I understand how to sleep, I set it to whatever time I want.

You often hear people say they are a morning person or a night owl etc. (perhaps you have believed or said something similar), but I know from personal experience that it isn't true.

You're neither, and you're both. By changing your behaviours, you can set your sleep to whatever time you want. And most of the time it comes, right on cue!

Sleep Knowledge 5
Insomnia and sleep deprivation are
not the same thing

Sleep deprivation is caused by a lack of opportunity to sleep and causes extreme drowsiness; the I-can't-keep-my-eyes-open feeling.

Somebody working for a week late into the night to meet a deadline and only giving themselves 5 hours a night to sleep would be somebody who will be experiencing short-term sleep deprivation and will struggle to keep themselves from falling asleep during the day.

Insomnia is not a lack of opportunity to sleep. If you take me as an example, I did not have a lack of opportunity to sleep – quite the opposite. I would sometimes spend 10, 11, 12 hours in bed trying to force sleep. I would be tired, anxious, stressed and fatigued during the day, but I never had the feeling that I could barely keep my eyes open and had to fight to stay awake.

When I had insomnia, I felt like I must be sleep deprived. Some nights it felt like I only slept for two hours a night or had no sleep whatsoever. However, while I felt like I was only sleeping for a couple of hours, the reality was very different.

Below is an excerpt from an article entitled '(Mis)Perception of Sleep in Insomnia: A Puzzle and a Resolution'. I will be providing a link to the entire article in the resource pages at the back of this book.

Mercer, Bootzin, and Lack (2002) compared the sleep perception of 14 patients with insomnia with 8 good sleepers. Sleep was monitored polysomnographically. When the participants were woken five minutes after the onset of Stage 2 sleep or during uninterrupted rapid eye movement (REM) sleep, patients with insomnia were more likely than the good sleepers to report experiencing wakefulness the moment just prior to being woken up. This finding applied to both the beginning and the end of the sleep period. Importantly, Mercer et al. (2002) also found that the laboratory measures of this tendency to interpret sleep as wakefulness correlated significantly with the discrepancy between subjective (sleep diary-defined) and objective (PSG-defined) sleep estimates based on 2 nights of home recordings ($r = .35–.83$). The latter finding suggests that the misperception of sleep exhibited by patients with insomnia may involve a tendency towards interpreting sleep as wakefulness. (Harvey and Tang 2012)

Thinking continues when we are sleeping, so it is common to think you are awake when you are asleep, and there is a considerable body of evidence to back this up.

When I spent 12 hours in bed trying to force sleep, I thought I was only sleeping 3 or maybe 4 hours a night, but I was sleeping longer.

The body needs a core amount of sleep, and it will find ways to get it. My sleep quality was very poor, and I was experiencing long periods of wakefulness as I lay there in my anxious state trying to force sleep. However, all the evidence pointed to the fact that I was sleeping longer than I thought and that I wasn't sleep deprived.

As I said in an earlier Sleep Knowledge section:

When objectively measured people with no sleep problems overestimate how much they sleep.

When objectively measured, people with insomnia underestimate how they sleep.

When I had insomnia and I first learnt that I was getting more sleep than I thought, despite all the evidence, I didn't believe it. 'You are wrong,' I thought. 'Perhaps this is true for everyone else, but I feel dreadful. I must be sleep deprived.'

Perhaps you think something similar.

But I wasn't sleep deprived. I now know this for a fact. And when you read my sleep window experience (a very powerful technique where you spend less time in bed), you will see for yourself why I am so confident in this assertion. But the proof is always in the pudding, so later on in the book I will teach you how you can set your own sleep window.

After you have experienced the sleep window yourself, you will also be able to say, 'Insomnia is not the same as sleep deprivation' as confidently as I do!

6

Islands and Tipis

America. Perhaps insomnia isn't a fan of long-haul flights and prefers to have its tea in the cupboard rather than coffee in the closet. After our ski season, I had a short-term job. It was on an island in the San Juans, situated right on the border of Vancouver. Paradise, golden beaches and clear, blue waters inhabited by orca whales.

The San Juan Islands are more or less exclusively owned by the wealthiest people on the entire planet, and mega yachts are as common as popcorn on a cinema floor.

It was pretty much a closed toy shop, a billionaire's playground, but slap bang in the middle of the excess and opulence, sticking both fingers up at Bill and Jeff as it hogged the swing set was Johns Island. A not-for-profit Native American camp built on the Lhaq'temish (Lummi) tribe's ancestral lands.

I was on Johns Island to teach theatre, build dug-out canoes, cook on campfires and fish for salmon. I arrived at the camp a week early to build a stage, clear out the log cabins, get firewood prepared for the wood-fired shower blocks and repair and set up the accommodation – Native American Sioux tipis, fifty in total.

Johns Island was a beautiful place with a beautiful purpose and philosophy, and for a brief period, it also gave me what I was seeking. Sleep.

For the first four weeks of being on the island, I slept. Better than I had for years. At the time, I didn't know why. I do now.

Sleeping in my tipi with only a few millimetres of canvas between me and nature, I could hear and feel the breath of the world. It would lull me to sleep every night, and every morning I would get up with the breakfast bell at 7 am. I would get up, get light and get active, and every night without fail I seemed to sleep.

I've cracked it, I thought. I need to be in tune with nature, and then my insomnia will be a thing of the past. So when I get home, I'm going off-grid, growing veggies and showering in streams. It's my lifestyle that is preventing me from sleeping, I thought. I just need a radical overhaul; it will be worth it for sleep. I'm going to do it!

I was ecstatic. The anxious thoughts before bed were still there, but with a month of evidence that I could sleep reasonably well, they were peripheral and in the background. For the first time in my life, I thought I had cracked the mystery of sleep. When things are going well and you are living the perfect life for you, you sleep. When things are going badly and you're not, you don't. Simple!

But predictably, without a true understanding of why I had been sleeping well, this brief spell of 'normal sleep' came to an abrupt end.

One night I couldn't sleep. Why? I had no idea. I just couldn't. And that one night of poor sleep simply wasn't acceptable to me, not when I knew and feared what it could become. So being the problem solving and survival machine that it is, my brain had to know why that poor night of sleep occurred to prevent it from ever happening again.

And why had it happened? Despite searching and obsessing about the reason for the whole of the following day, I couldn't come up with a concrete answer, but I had a few theories.

Perhaps I stayed up too late into the evening playing music, or perhaps I had had a stimulating conversation too late in the evening, and I was thinking about that. Maybe it was that run I went on only a few hours before bedtime that left me too energised. I enjoyed doing those things, but were they worth a sleepless night? Definitely not!

Sleep is a fragile thing I said to myself, and I must do everything I possibly can to protect it!

So, the next night, I went to bed early, and I made sure I didn't repeat any of the same silly mistakes that had caused my insomnia.

Did sleep come the second night? No. Somehow, I had messed up I told myself. Before bedtime, despite trying my best, I must have done something wrong.

The third night, I redoubled my efforts and was even more careful to avoid doing anything wrong to protect my sleep. And again, no sleep.

After the third night in a row, I resigned myself to failure. I thought I had cracked it. I thought by sleeping out in a tipi, on an island, surrounded by orcas, I had found the magic formula specific to me that allowed me to control sleep, but yet again I hadn't.

I had run 10,000 miles away, but, yet again, insomnia had hunted me down and brought its two friends along – behaviour changes and hyperarousal!

Sleep Knowledge 6
Active and avoidance sleep efforts

I learnt the terms active and avoidance sleep efforts from my sleep tutor Daniel Erichsen.

Hot baths, kiwi fruits, meditation, relaxation. These are some of the active methods I have taken in the past to force sleep.

Did they help? No.

Let's take warm baths as an example of an active sleep effort.

If you don't sleep well after taking a warm bath, you've failed. You feel more and more disheartened because no matter what you try, you can't make yourself sleep. But you are desperate to sleep, so you move on to the next active sleep effort or adapt the current one (perhaps if I put lavender bubble bath or Epsom salts in next time maybe then it will work).

If you do sleep well after a warm bath, then that's great, right? You have slept. All you need to do is always take warm baths before bed, and then you will never have insomnia ever again.

But what happens if, for example, you stay in a hotel that doesn't have a bathtub? Or maybe it has a bathtub, but you worry the maid will come in halfway through and be somewhat underwhelmed.

That's not very relaxing.

And maybe the bath's not as big as the one you have at home. And hot baths only **make** you sleep if you can lie flat in them. If your knees poke out, that's no good. What gives you the audacity to think you will be able to sleep after taking a warm bath if your knees poke out in front of an underwhelmed maid? (Perhaps you'd better cancel that trip away after all.)

And what happens if you have the perfect maid-free warm bath with your knees fully submerged and the right brand of lavender bubble bath, Epsom salts and scented candles, but it doesn't work, and you don't sleep? What then?

If hot baths, kiwi fruit and meditation make you sleep, what does that mean? That means you can't sleep without them; that means you have lost the innate ability to sleep that everybody has. That means there is something wrong with you, and you need something external to force you to sleep.

What you have done is placed your confidence in the hot bath, kiwi fruit or meditation technique at the expense of your confidence in your innate ability to sleep.

But have you lost your innate ability to sleep? Did the hot bath make you sleep, or were you just sleepy and, because you believed that hot baths make you sleep, you were less anxious (hyperaroused) about not sleeping?

Now does all this mean you can never enjoy a hot bath (meditation, kiwi fruit) before bed ever again? No, definitely not. If you like hot baths and you find them relaxing, then that's great.

It's not the action that steals your confidence; it's the intention.

Hot baths cannot make you sleep. Every time you have slept after taking one (or after doing a relaxation technique or meditating ...), you have slept all by yourself. You slept because the body needs sleep, and you were feeling sleepy.

If you are sleepy, and you are not hyperaroused you will sleep.

Now we have active sleep efforts covered, let's move on.

I would like to, but I can't play music before bed. I can't have stimulating conversations before bed. I can't go for a run too soon before bed.

I would like to, but I can't eat late in a restaurant, go on a holiday and stay in a hotel in case my knees stick out, go kickboxing, roller skating or meet my friends for a drink ...

All of the above are **avoidance** sleep efforts.

Indeed, going to a running group late in the evening before going to bed may have a slight effect on sleep. So can meeting up with friends and having a couple of deep mugs of ale. So can a whole host of other things too numerous to mention.

Normal sleepers will also typically sleep better in their own bed than at a hotel.

But do they not go on a weekend break away, not join a running group or not meet up with their friends for drinks in the evening in case they don't sleep as well?

Lots of things that you avoid may affect sleep in the short term. But treating sleep as though it is fragile and needs to be pro-tected will make you worry and obsess about sleep and have a negative impact on your sleep over the long term.

Not only will it have a negative impact on your sleep. It will also have a negative impact on your life, your health and your happiness.

Active sleep efforts erode your confidence.

Avoidance sleep efforts erode your agency. (Agency is the feeling of having control over your life.)

7

Sleeping Tablets

I was in America, in paradise with the most beautiful people from all corners of the world, people who were just like me. Odd.

Before my insomnia returned, I was happy to be there. But now things were different. The place was the same, the people were the same, but spending the whole day worrying and obsessing about sleep I didn't feel like I was properly there anymore. Now it felt like the colour was drained out of everything and I was watching from afar.

I just want to be home, I said to myself. Home, where I don't have to get up for the breakfast bell at 7 am every single day. Home, where there are weekends and lie-ins. Home, where I can finally get some sleep!

Marooned on an island, I felt utterly lost and alone. But then I heard the unmistakable sound of a cockerel being flung against a chainsaw, and I knew that I wasn't.

Crystal. There was no mistaking that laugh.

Crystal was from New Jersey. She was tiny, with an aquiline nose and a razor-sharp wit.

'Brown hair zig zagged across her face and a look of half surprise, Like a fox caught in the headlights there was animal in her eyes.' (I stole that line from songwriter Richard Thompson as nothing could ever describe Crystal better.)

I told Crystal about how I hadn't slept.

'Sleeping tablets,' she screeched. (Crystal never said anything, ever, she screeched, laughed and guffawed, but she never said anything.) 'I can't sleep without them.'

On Crystal's advice and after a short doctor's appointment, only a few hours later, I had a pack of twenty-eight Zolpidem sleeping pills in my hand.

That night I cracked one through the foil, washed it down and lay in my tipi. I didn't for a second believe it would work. Nothing else had. But within 30 minutes or so, my anxiety seemed to melt, my thoughts fractured, and I was out cold, gone.

I was down for 7 hours or so. After four years of searching, I had found what seemed to be a miracle cure for my problem.

Guaranteed sleep in a little capsule. I didn't have to change or do anything. I took the tablet, and I could sleep, just like everybody else. What's more, I could set sleep to my schedule. Need to get up at 7 am. No problem. Take the tablet at 11.30 pm, sleep would come at 12 am, and then I would get 7 hours of sleep, guaranteed.

It was such a relief. I felt for the first time since my insomnia that I had complete control over my sleep. I was still forcing sleep, but the difference was, this time, the force I was using was a sleeping pill. And it worked.

I was so happy. Well, I would have been if it hadn't been for the gnawing feeling that I tried to push away. I was sleeping, or I certainly felt like I was sleeping. And for 7 hours a night. But the next day I wouldn't have known it. The next day I felt low and irritable and had no energy. Not good, I said to myself, but much better than it was surely …

I felt better than when I didn't take a sleeping tablet and only slept for 1 or 2 hours. I felt even worse the next day then. What's more, Zolpidem also offered me something other than just sleep – certainty.

Without the tablet, when 12 am came round, I had to play sleep Russian Roulette (will I sleep tonight or won't I?). With it I didn't. I took it, and I was gone. I wasn't getting the sleep that I wanted, but what I was getting was the certainty of escaping the night. And that, in and of itself, was enough.

Sleep Knowledge 7
Doctor knows best?

First of all, how do sleeping tablets work?

They don't make you sleep. Nothing makes you sleep except your sleep drive. Sleeping pills work through sedation and make you unable to form the complex thoughts that make you hyperaroused.

They can also work through 'delegation'. In the moment you take the pill, you have delegated the work of sleeping. You're no longer responsible, you're no longer trying and, when you make no effort to sleep – you sleep!

With Zolpidem, it would usually take 30 minutes or so before I felt its effect, but I have lost count of the number of times I fell asleep within 5 minutes of taking it!

Now that we have covered how sleeping pills work, this is the part where I make you feel guilty about taking them, right? No. You take sleeping pills? Of course you do! I did too.

Your body is doing something you don't want and can't control. Sleeping pills offer you a sense of control, a sense of certainty. If, like me, everything else you have tried up to now to give yourself that certainty hasn't worked, when you find something that does, you will grasp it with both hands.

I don't take Zolpidem any more, and I assume, like me, you want healthy, long-term, natural sleep. But what happens when you go to the doctor's to get it?

You get sleeping tablets.

Or you get sleep-hygiene advice. And you go back a second time. And you get more sleep-hygiene advice. And you go back a third time, and then eventually get some sleeping tablets for short-term use – but on the understanding that they are awful for you, and addictive, and that you really ought not to be taking them.

And by the way, did you know that your bedroom should be cool and that you shouldn't drink caffeine after 3 pm? So if you are sleeping in your sauna and taking espresso shots to the eyeballs, stop it!

If you have been to the doctor's for your insomnia, how did it make you feel?

Only being prescribed sleeping tablets and being given advice I had followed a thousand times already made me feel that my insomnia couldn't be cured.

They are doctors. They have studied their entire lives, and insomnia is widespread, so surely they know everything there is to know about it.

And if the only thing they can tell me is sleep hygiene and offer me sleeping tablets, that means I can't sleep on my own and that there must be something very wrong with me.

But there isn't. And on this occasion, your doctor doesn't know best.

Doctors must have a terrible time of it. They want to help people, and they will see hundreds, if not thousands of insomniacs throughout their career.

But do you know the average amount of training a UK medical student devotes to sleep medicine during the whole of their 5–7 year training? 1.5 hours (Romisewski et al. 2020).

And that's not 1.5 hours devoted to insomnia. That includes (but is not limited to) respiratory sleep conditions such as sleep apnoea, sleep disorders in psychiatry, parasomnias, hypersomnias and sleep disorders in children.

You are only a third of the way through this book, but I guarantee you already know considerably more about insomnia than the vast majority of doctors. So back yourself, you've got this!

If, then, you are taking sleeping pills, I'm not going to tell you to stop taking them. And if you do decide to stop taking them, always do it under your doctor's care and advice.

I am, however, going to tell you that shouldn't feel any guilt about it. None whatsoever. Because when, like me, you first started taking sleeping pills, you were doing the best you could on the information and limited knowledge you had at the time.

You're also doing the best you can right now because, just by reading this book, you have taken the first step to slowly but surely get to a place where you will feel safe and confident enough in your own innate ability to sleep that you can do it all by yourself!

8

Jobs in the City

On returning home from America, I hoped that I would sleep. I went to America in the hope that I would sleep, and I came back from America in the hope that I would sleep.

Pushing myself from pillar to post trying to find the perfect life and lifestyle to magically sleep was becoming a habit.

I wasn't, however, going to get a perfect life, not yet anyway. I returned home from America at the age of 23 with no money, no house and no prospects. So, like everyone else, Claire and I moved to the city.

We both got jobs. Mine was a proper one, a well-paid indoors one where everything was streamlined and monochrome.

I went to huddles in think tanks and used phrases like 'projected outcomes' and 'quarterly reports'. I was part of a dynamic forward-thinking company which sold something that nobody really wanted or needed and that I was expected to pretend to be excited about.

I shouldn't have been there. I didn't belong. I knew it, and so did everyone else.

It was here that I had the worst episode of insomnia I have ever had in my life. In America, when insomnia struck, I had a get-out. In the UK, I didn't. I could get hold of sleeping tablets, but not like I could in America. Fourteen, every 3 months. (They are addictive, don't you know?) I could take one a week (although that changed later on in my insomnia, when I started taking sleeping tablets far more frequently).

That was it.

So, night after night I slept for one, possibly two, hours a night (or so I thought at the time, but as you and I have already learnt from the Sleep Knowledge section entitled 'Insomnia is not the same as sleep deprivation' that wasn't the case).

I spent the days desperate to be in bed. I spent the nights desperate to be out of it.

The anxiety was overwhelming; everything felt colourless, out of control and sped-up, like watching the blur of a grey, concrete landscape through the window of a speeding train.

I had an excellent job, so I had to be there. Didn't I? No, I was choosing to be there.

It was my choice. And it was my choice to leave. We were in the middle of the 2008 crash. It was a good job, and I quit.

I hadn't quit anything before; what did that say about me? Was it a good thing? In retrospect, most definitely. At the time, good, bad, who knows?

But it did leave me with a problem. Where will I go? What will I do? I thought about that for a while as I drove my little red

Ford Fiesta along the motorway. At first I was consumed with regret, fear, shame and guilt about my failure. But all of a sudden, a huge smile appeared on my face when I realised I could now go anywhere and do anything.

That night I went home happy and relaxed. As soon as my head hit the pillow, I slept. I slept the clock the whole way round. 12 hours. Probably the deepest and longest sleep of my life. I woke up reborn. But I also woke up convinced of the fallacy that it is the events that occur in my life that dictate whether or not I can sleep. If I can control them, then I can control my sleep.

Sleep Knowledge 8
The events in your life do not control your sleep

Get a different job, and I will sleep. Move to another city, and I will sleep. When my son, daughter, husband, wife, mum, dad, dog, next-door neighbour stops doing this and starts doing that instead, I will sleep.

Yes, as we have covered earlier in the book, stressful or distressing events can trigger a short-term sleep problem, but they are not what causes insomnia.

I thought I could control sleep by trying to get everything in my life to align perfectly. It's true that I did sleep better after I quit my job in the city, but I still never slept like a 'normal sleeper' and never had a healthy relationship with sleep until I learnt how to sleep.

During my sleep course (as you will read later in the book), I was going through the most challenging time I had ever had in my entire life. But, armed with the right sleep knowledge, I slept better than I had ever done since the onset of my insomnia.

Perhaps you know somebody who is unhappy in their work or in their relationship, somebody who has financial pressure or is going through a bereavement or an incredibly distressing time who more or less still sleeps reasonably well most nights.

Probably, and that is because it is not the events in their life that control their sleep. Just as it is not the events in your life that control yours.

9

Nursing and Tipis

Neither my partner nor I liked city life, and we both hated our jobs. So what would we do now that we were knee-deep in a global recession and penniless but were free to do anything?

First, off we moved to a tiny village on the Welsh border. Our 'house' was a 300-year-old cottage. It had no loft insulation, broken windowpanes and no heating.

Have you ever seen a mouse squeeze itself under the crack of a door? It's remarkable what they can do. The mice we had at our cottage didn't need to do any squeezing; in fact, the drafts under the door were so vast, I'm sure next door's cat could have followed them.

It would have been freezing at the best of times, but to add a little extra spice, we moved in the Autumn of 2009, 3 months before the coldest winter on record, when we would regularly see temperatures down to minus 20.

We wore full ski gear inside the house, salopettes, thermals, ski coats and gloves during this winter. And if we wanted to flush the toilet, we first had to boil a kettle to melt the ice in the cistern.

Our cottage was situated on the end of a terrace at the end of a no-through street with a pallet-making factory behind a chain-link fence to the side of us. Pete, our landlord lived next door.

Pete was in his seventies, with light-blue eyes, gunmetal hair and skeletal, nervous hands, and always wore dusty blue overalls. Pete's favourite thing to say was how he 'worked hard and got on' and that he would work six days a week, half-days on Sundays.

I know why. Pete was sadly inflicted with OCD and would have to repeat everything he did multiple times. It would take him 10 minutes to lock a door as he would have to check each lock over and over again. If outside, I would occasionally hear him through the door repeating to himself 'bolt lock, door lock, bolt lock, door lock etc. etc.' Now I look back on it, I can see many similarities between the rituals Pete would have to go through during his daily life and those that I put myself through to force sleep. I'm sure Pete's seemed as necessary and logical to him as my own did to me.

Pete would also keep an eye on us constantly.

The combination of a harassing landlord and a hovel of a house most people wouldn't have put up with, and they would have been justified to think that way, but we had no choice. It was the cheapest house by far that we could find, and we had no money.

Claire was training to be a nurse, so didn't have an income, and I was pouring everything that I had left over from my job (working with adults and children with autism and learning disabilities) into setting up a new business.

I based it on my time spent in America. Native American tipi hire with real wood fires. It was a stupid idea, especially as we were in the middle of a recession, and virtually everybody I explained my idea to told me so. So I stopped telling people and did it anyway.

In the first year of doing it – pouring in every spare penny I had to buy as many tipis as possible and with a bit of a ropey website – they were proved right. I didn't even break even. But in the second year, glamping suddenly became the most fashionable thing on the planet, business exploded, and I was catapulted headfirst into the most fantastic world of adventure.

I worked on TV and film sets. I set tipis up at and got invited to weddings so lavish that one I attended had booked zoo animals and imported an entire water park to keep the children entertained. For the adults? Show jumping and a formation MiG jet fly over!

Once I was setting up a tipi in the garden on bonfire night trying to work out how to get away from Radiohead's Thom Yorke so I could ring Kate Moss's secretary to arrange a booking for the following weekend.

During the week, I was falling through the floorboards of my dilapidated cottage, and at the weekends I was being cooked dinner by TV chefs and brought cups of tea by supermodels. It was like I had found a way to move between parallel universes. It was bizarre.

It was also a solid time for myself and my partner. Trite as it sounds, we were both living authentically. She was working towards a purpose she loved, and I had found something that gave me the excitement and variety that I craved. It was the strongest we had ever been. But it turns out we were in the eye of the storm before the winds of complacency and neglect would rip through our relationship.

And there was something new with my sleep. I was finding it quite a lot easier now to fall asleep, and, for probably a good few months, I was sleeping better than I had for a long time because of it.

My insomnia before had always been trouble falling asleep, but I was usually OK once I was there. But I had pulled a muscle in my neck, and I was waking up due to the fact that I was uncomfortable.

At first, I didn't think much of it and would fall asleep quickly. But I started to notice that I always seemed to wake up at the same time. It was like I could set my watch by it, and the more I noticed it, the more of a problem it became, and the more of a problem it became, the more I noticed it, and the time it took me to get back to sleep seemed to get longer and longer. And it wasn't the stiff neck any more that was doing it, that had passed, but the 3 am night-time awakening remained.

Sleep Knowledge 9
The stages of sleep

Sleep has been traditionally divided into four categories: awake, light, deep, and REM sleep. Each stage runs for approximately 90 minutes.

Deep sleep is more common in the first half of the night, and REM sleep is more common in the second half of the night. It is therefore normal for sleep to be lighter during the second half of the night. Because sleep runs in cycles, it is also normal to wake many times throughout the night and to fall back to sleep again.

As we age, it is typical to become more aware of being awake as we have more conditions that can interfere with sleep (medication and physical and mental ailments).

It is normal to wake up many times throughout the night – everybody does – but a person with insomnia will typically have trouble going back to sleep again and will often blame the insomnia on the medication or the ailment.

But is the medication or the ailment the cause of insomnia?

Below is an excerpt from a personal communication with my sleep tutor Daniel Erichsen.

This may surprise you, but all humans wake up multiple times … every hour! It is part of the safety system where we wake up briefly and we become aware of sounds and the environment in general. And if everything seems safe we resume sleeping shortly after.

So waking up in itself is a completely normal part of sleeping. When you wake up, become aware of being awake and then it takes a long time to fall back asleep again, now that's a different story.

The most important thing here is again to recognize that it is not the waking up that is a problem, but rather how we respond to it.

Someone who generally speaking sleeps well will wake up, roll around, go back to sleep and not even remember the following day. And this is because being awake is not a threat for them. Being awake is not something they respond to.

When you have had trouble sleeping on the other hand, being awake at night is something that the brain has started thinking of as a threat or a problem. And because it's trying to keep you safe, the brain is now looking out for wakefulness.

So when you become awake, even briefly, the brain reacts to this by waking up further in a misguided attempt at keeping you safe!

So what to do when this is happening? Well again, befriending wakefulness is the way. And two other things are really good as well.

Firstly, resist any urge to know what time it is! This is a very powerful way of letting go of attempts at controlling sleep.

Second, don't argue with reality! Simply acknowledge that you are awake just like you would acknowledge that it's 72 degrees outside. This is not resignation, it's simply taking note of a fact.

This doesn't seem like rocket science but when you simply acknowledge that you're awake and no longer try to change this forcefully, you are doing something super helpful: letting go of attempts at trying to make yourself sleep. And with less attempts at trying to make sleep happen; with less pressure, the easier sleep happens. (Erichsen, personal communication, 16 January 2021)

10

Devon and Bell Tents

In 2012 Claire and I relocated to Devon. Here we bought a tiny fisherman's cottage, complete with brown dalmatian on the second-hand sofa. It was beautiful, watertight and warm! Claire was now a qualified nurse, and the tipi hire was going well. The days of poverty and living in a freezing medieval hovel were over.

We surfed in the evenings and sat by the wood burner at night – paradise! We married in 2015. We danced to a ceilidh band for hours; all our favourite people in the world were at the small venue by the river to celebrate our love and life together. Unfortunately, it didn't last.

Shortly after our marriage, I set up a new business. The tipi hire business was fun and adventurous, but it was hard: seventy-hour weeks, rain, storms, heavy lifting, hours of motorway driving. I knew everything there was to know about tents, so my new business was importing and selling canvas bell tents. The first year was a challenge. But by the second year, it worked. Too well.

It was easy. I woke to an inbox stuffed with orders. I rang the courier company, and they shipped the tents out. On one order for Glastonbury Festival, I made as much money in 5 minutes as I had working a hundred sixteen-hour shifts at my job with children with autism that I had continued alongside my tipi hire business. I should have been happy, but I wasn't.

It was meaningless. It was fun for the first year when I was struggling and determined to make it work. I had money, but I had no challenge, no ambition and no adventure.

Derek Trotter said it best in the final scene of *Only Fools and Horses* after he had achieved his dream of becoming a multi-millionaire: 'The chase is ... finished. The hunt is over. What am I going to do now? Learn to play golf? ... I want to feel like I used to feel, all eager and alive ... I want something exciting to happen.'

I suppose what I was selling was the means for people to get back and reconnect with nature. They are magical tents and incredibly relaxing to spend time in. But could I keep on selling bell tents forever? Was it my raison d'être, the thing in life that makes all other hardships worthwhile? Something that I always wanted to improve on, read and learn everything I possibly could about to try to do my absolute best for people like I am trying to do now as I write this book for you? No. It wasn't any of those things.

In his book *Tribe: On Homeconing and Belonging*, Sebastian Junger writes: 'Humans don't mind hardship, in fact they **thrive** on it; what they mind is not feeling necessary. Modern society has perfected the art of making people not feel necessary.'

I wasn't helping anybody apart from myself, and I didn't feel necessary.

And there was another problem. The business more or less ran itself, so every day was like a weekend, which meant I could indulge in my insomnia more than ever.

There was no need for a routine, so my learnt behaviours of forcing sleep and waking late in the afternoon could be indulged. I was spending 13, 14, 15 hours in bed, forcing and wrestling with sleep, eventually managing it when everybody else was beginning their day.

The time I was compelled to spend in the torture chamber was growing month by month, but I had to sleep, so I felt like I had to be there. And as my time in bed grew, so too did my anxiety, fear and frustration about being in bed.

But what to do? If only there were a relaxation technique or way to make sleep happen. Well, luckily, the next sleep section will help you with that!

Sleep Knowledge 10
Relaxation techniques and the illusion of failure

I'm guessing with all the sleep knowledge you have gained so far, your anxiety around sleep has already started to lesson,

But what can you do in bed to make yourself sleep if it just isn't coming?

Well, the breathing exercise below is one that you can try. It is not traditionally used for sleep in its current form, but the better you learn it, the easier it will be to adapt so it can be utilised for your insomnia.

I want you to follow the steps exactly. If you don't do it perfectly, it won't work. Use a pleasant soothing voice to do it with. Morgan Freeman is a good bet, but check with him first that you don't have to pay royalties.

1) Close your eyes and take three deep slow breaths. Visualise a ball of warm, white light. Breathe that white light down into your chest and your heart chakra.

2) Now, with another breath in, suck that white light down into your coccyx (the coccyx is often forgotten about in these breathing exercises, so I thought I'd give it a little treat).

3) Push that warm, white light down through your legs and into your feet and repeat after me, 'I will make my hair blue,' and again, 'I will make my hair blue,' and again, 'I will make my hair blue.' Don't worry if you don't have any hair like me; give yourself some (I've always wanted a mullet), and then make it blue.

4) Repeat ten more times.

After one final breath out, stand up, take a wander and look in the bathroom mirror.

Check you out with your feet all aglow, smiley happy face complete with a head of lovely blue hair starring back at you!

Oh, it hasn't worked? Well, in that case you have failed.

Do what I just said every day for 2, 3, 4, 5 hours until you eventually succeed. And if it doesn't work, you're not doing it properly, not doing it long enough or you're not trying hard enough.

Sound familiar? Nobody can make their hair blue by using breathing techniques. Nobody can get to the moon on a skateboard. Nobody can force themselves to feel hungry by sitting at the dinner table and repeating to themselves, 'I feel hungry. I feel hungry,' and nobody can force themselves to sleep using relaxation techniques if they are not already sleepy.

Relaxation can reduce anxiety, but it cannot make you sleep. It is impossible. There is not one person on the planet who can do it.

Now, I'm not saying don't meditate in the evening, don't use breathing exercises, or stop doing yoga in the evenings. Relaxation techniques, meditation, sitting with a nice cup of yogi tea or reading a book are great at helping you let go of the day.

They are also great for your well-being and amazing for helping you reduce anxiety. But if, like I used to, you are using these techniques to try to force sleep when you are not sleepy, you are fighting a losing battle because it is not possible.

Any time you are in bed scrunching yourself into a ball and becoming angry with yourself that you can't force yourself to sleep, any time you are taking your hot baths, kiwi fruits, supplements or indeed engaging in any activity with the express intention of making yourself sleep, I want you to picture yourself scrunching your face up and trying to force your hair to turn blue.

Don't get me wrong. It's OK that you've done it in the past. I did it too. But now you know what you are doing, please, stop being such a turnip!

11

Supplements and Kiwis

As my insomnia gradually worsened, so too did my obsession with it. I would spend hours every day sitting in front of the laptop searching for different methods, hoping beyond hope to find that magic relaxation or breathing technique to make me sleep.

I tried them all – acupuncture, meditation, reflexology – the list is endless. And they didn't work, so I went on a hunt for something else: supplements and sleep-inducing food.

GABA. I looked it up and studied it in detail. That's it, I thought. I can't sleep because I have a physical problem with my brain. It doesn't produce GABA. That must be the reason.

I would then immediately order a bottle and, while waiting for it to arrive, spend hours researching the brain chemical:

> GABA (Gamma-aminobutyric acid) the chief inhibitory neurotransmitter in the developmentally mature mammalian central nervous system.

Wait! I'm a mature mammalian too! That must be it!

I would take a look at the chemical formula and try to know everything I could about it. It arrived. I took it, and nothing.

Still the same obsession and anxiety, only now ever so slightly worse as it was just another thing to add to the laundry list of things that didn't work.

So I would go back to the internet and research GABA some more and come across the following information: 'There is conflicting information that the supplement GABA doesn't cross the blood-brain barrier.'

OK, so that is the problem, I would tell myself. I have no idea what the blood-brain barrier is, but it sounds fancy, so let's see what else I can take that does cross the blood-brain barrier. L-Theanine elevates levels of GABA as well as serotonin and dopamine!

Right, so maybe it is a GABA problem. Or perhaps it is a serotonin or dopamine problem.

So I would order a box of L-theanine. And, nothing. Into the wicker basket it went.

5HTP, magnolia bark, ashwagandha, magnesium, tryptophan, CBD, valerian, jujube. None of them worked, but I kept taking them anyway. Every night I would chug down a massive cocktail mixed with grapefruit juice, kiwi fruit and cherries. (Apparently grapefruit juice makes everything more effective, kiwis increase serotonin, and cherries – who knows why I took them, but I did!)

And nothing. Always nothing. All it served to do was fuel my obsession and anxiety around sleep, and the more it did that, the more insomnia stretched its bony fingers into my long days and fitful nights.

And as my obsession grew, so did my avoidance methods to try to protect sleep.

I can't go surfing in the evenings because if I do that, I'll be so energised I won't sleep.

I can't visit a friend and stay over at their house because if I do that, I won't sleep.

I can't see a live band or play my saxophone at an open mic because if I do that, I won't sleep. I can't, I can't, I can't.

Slowly but surely, I stripped the things I loved from life in the pursuit of something that was always out of my reach.

And the more I did, the further away it got from me, and the further away I got from myself and everyone and everything around me.

I was detached. Numb. Physically and emotionally.

My confidence and self-esteem shot gone. And that's when the character assassination started in earnest. I would say to myself, 'You used to be funny; you used to be intelligent, adventurous, confident, fearless; you used to skydive, surf, work hard, have an amazing business and enjoy life. But now, look at you.'

'You are not like that anymore.'

'And you never will be again.'

Sleep Knowledge 11
Can supplements or food be used to cure insomnia?

You are about halfway through this book, so you know the answer to that already. No.

Take kiwi fruit, for example. I first heard about kiwi fruit curing insomnia on a documentary by Michael Mosley. The science behind how kiwi fruit can help you sleep is that they contain serotonin which is then converted to melatonin.

There was a research study conducted in China entitled 'Effect of kiwifruit consumption on sleep quality in adults with sleep problems'. Here the participants each ate two kiwi fruit before bed. The results? Waking time after sleep onset and sleep-onset latency were decreased.

Excellent news. So kiwi fruits do work.

No. If they worked, insomnia wouldn't exist.

You'd go to your doctor. They would hand you a fruit bowl and tell you not to drive or operate heavy machinery. Problem solved.

Taking two kiwi fruit every night before bed when you have a chronic insomnia issue will make things worse as they will only serve to increase the obsession, rituals and desire for sleep.

Maybe if somebody with no trouble sleeping were to have a couple of kiwi fruit before bed, they might get a few more minutes' sleep, but are kiwi fruit the cure for a chronic, long-term problem?

You know the answer to that too, otherwise you wouldn't be here.

There is evidence that sweet potatoes can help people lose weight, but will eating a sweet potato a day help somebody who wants to lose 20 stone but who makes no other behaviour and lifestyle changes?

Kiwi fruit, supplements, cherries don't work, and you know they don't work because you have probably tried them, or something like them, already.

What are kiwi fruit and supplements? That's right, active sleep efforts. And we know where that leads! That leads to you sit-ting in the bath with your knees poking out, in front of an un-derwhelmed maid, scrunching your face up and trying to turn your hair blue. It's not a good look.

12

Divorce and Depression

I was broken. I was done, and I wanted out. I thought I had found a way. One day a pop-up appeared on my computer screen for an online test for depression.

I ticked nearly all the boxes. It wasn't surprising. I had stripped all the things I loved from my life. I had a business that gave me no sense of purpose, and I had a relationship that had crumbled to dust around me. I had had insomnia for twenty years, but depression? How long had I had that? Two years? Three? I don't know.

I should have seen the warning signs earlier, but of course, as Homer said, 'After the event, even a fool is wise.'

That's it, I thought. That's why I can't sleep. Depression causes insomnia. It is well documented.

So I went back to the doctor's, and this time instead of sleeping pills, I had a new prescription for antidepressants. And I took them. And nothing.

No improvement in my depression. No improvement in my insomnia. Nothing.

That was a hard blow. I had pinned my hopes on these tablets working for me. But like everything else, they didn't. I was distraught, but if I thought things were bad now, they were about to get worse.

My wife and I separated and started divorce proceedings in 2018. It was as amicable and friendly as possible. No backbiting, no hiring lawyers to squabble over money; we were leaving each other's lives, but despite everything, I think there was still enough love and care there that we wanted the best for each other.

Insomnia did play a large part in the breakdown of our marriage. And a lot was my fault, but of course, there are two people in a relationship.

When it comes to relationships, the Vietnamese monk Thich Nhat Hanh said it far better than I ever could: 'You must love in such a way that the person you love feels free.'

Perhaps neither of us got that quite right.

Separation forces you to confront the things you have buried. What I had buried was my biggest fear that behind my smile was somebody who wasn't good enough and that one day I would be found out. During times of self-doubt I still feel like this.

I feel this fear is something we all share to some degree. We mask it in different ways, sometimes positively by pursuing career and status, and sometimes negatively through addictions and destructive behaviours. Still, I feel at least to some degree, we all share this.

This fear is something that afflicts and unites us all. When a relationship has crumbled and everything is uncertain, you have no choice but to look this fear in the eye. And I believe how you respond to this determines how well or how badly you ultimately move on from it.

As well as my marriage, I lost my best friend during the divorce. I worked with him during the winter as a tree surgeon, so that work went too.

My business also failed, mostly from market forces but partly from neglect. Struggling to pay the mortgage, I moved into my camper van for a while.

Divorce was the hardest time of my life, but trite as it sounds, now that I am through it, it was the best thing that ever happened, and I wouldn't change it for the world.

Sleep Knowledge 12
Insomnia as a primary condition

As per the previous Sleep Knowledge section, doctors only receive a median of 1.5 hours of sleep medicine training.

Anxiety, PTSD, depression ... When you go to the doctors, they will often treat insomnia as a secondary condition to the primary one.

As happened in my case. I had depression. Depression was seen as the primary condition, and insomnia as the secondary. My insomnia was a symptom of my depression.

But is this the case? Are there people with anxiety, depression or PTSD who do not have chronic insomnia? And are their people with physical ailments like arthritis who also do not have insomnia?

My depression exacerbated my insomnia, but I had had insomnia for years before my depression, so how could depression be perpetuating my insomnia?

Let's take as an example somebody in acute pain for a period of time, which can often lead to a sleep problem. But what if, through the right medication, surgery etc., the pain is relieved but that person still has insomnia? If that is the case, then insomnia was not a symptom of the acute pain.

I am about to show you the steps I took to walk away from insomnia, but before I do, suppose we review the Sleep Knowledge sections up to now. Your insomnia is not unique. Insomnia is a primary condition, and sleeping tablets will not cure it. It doesn't matter what triggered your insomnia; your behaviours and thought patterns perpetuate it. Sleep is a natural process driven by the sleep drive, which can be masked by hyperarousal. Sleeping tablets do not make you sleep but may erode your confidence in your innate ability to sleep. You don't need 8 hours of sleep. It is normal to wake up multiple times throughout the night. Insomnia and sleep deprivation are not the same thing. Your life events don't control your insomnia. Active and avoidance sleep efforts exacerbate the problem, and you can't use diet and supplements to overcome insomnia. Just as it is impossible to turn your hair blue, it is impossible to make yourself sleep by using relaxation techniques!

So how do you overcome it? Well, for the remainder of this book, I'm going to show you how to resolve your insomnia by showing you how I resolved mine!

13

Resolving My Insomnia Through CBT-I

I never truly believed that I could find a cure for insomnia. Not really. I had tried what I thought was everything but to no avail.

All I was hoping for was a slight improvement. With the right supplement, the right meditation, the right relaxation technique, maybe I could still find something that could at least work a bit. And it was then that I stumbled across CBT-I.

Why, in my twenty years of searching, had I not come across CBT-I before? The truth is I had. I had probably heard of it ten years or so ago, but I never took the first step to look more deeply into it.

Why? Well, firstly, by then I had tried so many different things. And the more things I tried, the deeper and deeper CBT-I got buried amongst all the other stuff that didn't work.

And that was what I initially thought CBT-I was, just another thing that wouldn't work. I had become jaded. I had lurched from one thing to the other only to come up against brick walls and dead ends. The more this happened, the less confident I became about actually finding something that would.

CBT-I also required an investment of time and energy. I was happy enough to do that for a supplement or relaxation technique that I knew wouldn't work because that was easy. Pop the pill. It doesn't work. Move onto the next pill. But CBT-I? That was an eight-week course, and why would I want to put myself through the torment of an eight-week course just to find yet another thing that doesn't work?

Secondly, I think the name has a lot to do with why I was so reluctant to try CBT-I.

Let's break down the name:

Cognitive

Excellent. That works, nothing wrong with that. One of the pillars that holds up and perpetuates insomnia (as I wrote about earlier in a Sleep Knowledge section) is obsessive thought patterns, anxiety and a conditioned response to the bed being a place of, at best, wakefulness and, at worst, torment.

You have trouble sleeping, so you worry and obsess about not sleeping (hyperarousal), and this worry and obsession give you greater trouble sleeping, which makes you more worried and obsessed about sleep. Rinse and repeat.

Behavior

Excellent. The other key component that perpetuates insomnia is your behaviours. You have trouble sleeping, so you try to catch up on sleep by napping or waking up late. You have more difficulty sleeping, so you go to bed earlier and earlier and spend more and more time in bed trying to force sleep, which creates more trouble.

So you try to force sleep through relaxation techniques, meditation, bizarre rituals (north end of the bed, south end etc.), and you have even more trouble sleeping, so you then change your whole life in order to try to force sleep.

These behaviours make sleeping even harder, which feeds anxiety, worry and obsession (the *cognitive* pillar of insomnia). The behaviours feed the cognition, and the cognition feeds the behaviours, until every night you munch down a big steamy pile of insomnia. Not good.

Therapy

Problem. Big problem. What images does therapy conjure up for you? For me, it's lying down on a couch and talking about my insomnia.

'Now, Joseph, if together we can work out what caused your insomnia, then together we can help you sleep.'

Or maybe, 'Oh, that's very interesting. How does insomnia make you feel?'

('Well, not great, if I'm honest.')

Or 'Tell me about how your marriage is going tits-up while I make reassuring nodding motions and raise my eyebrows and say things like "Go on," and "That must be very hard for you," for £6.72 a syllable.'

(If my therapist ever reads this, I should point out she was amazing and helped me loads in other ways, just not with this issue!)

I had already done therapy, and I had already added it to the list of things that didn't work.

For me, the word therapy was the culprit. What would I change it to? I don't know. But I know who would. Kentucky Unbridled Spirit. Now that's a slogan. Whoever came up with that, I would hire for the rebranding of CBT- I immediately.

Sleep Knowledge 13
What is CBT-I and how effective is it?

So how effective are the sleep knowledge and behaviour changes I am sharing with you now? There are percentage figures I could give you regarding effectiveness, but I'm not going to. Why not? Because no matter how impressive they are (and they are impressive – what I am sharing with you is scientifically proven to be the most effective treatment there is – nothing else comes close), you will probably think just as I thought: 'Yes, it can work for them, but I know for a fact, I will be in the small percentage who can't overcome their insomnia, as my insomnia is the worst insomnia on the planet!'

It's understandable to think like this, especially if, like me, you have tried so many other things. But thinking like this wasn't helpful to me, and probably won't be for you.

(If you really want to know a figure and how it is determined, I include a link to a scientific study by Mitchell et al. in the References that will provide this information.)

It's worth noting that the results of the study into the effectiveness of CBT-I include participants who did not make or continue with the behaviour changes (behaviour changes are not always easy – but so worth it!) as well as those who did not make the psychological leap to reach a point where they truly understood that there is nothing they can do to force sleep so that they were no longer worried or anxious about it. In a nutshell they never reached the point where they just simply stopped caring about sleep.

Insomnia boils down to two problems: one concerning the sleep drive and the other hyperarousal.

The purpose of this book is to help you overcome both.

So, in answer to how effective the knowledge of what I am sharing with you is, what I will say is what I have said already. Everybody on the planet needs to sleep, just like everybody on the planet needs to drink. If you follow the behaviour changes that build a strong, regulated sleep drive and you reach a point where you are no longer anxious or worried about sleep (you are not hyperaroused), you will sleep. Everybody will.

If you are sleepy and you are not hyperaroused, you will sleep.

No exceptions! That one sentence is what this whole book boils down to.

What, then, is CBT-I?

Cognitive intervention

Sleep knowledge forms the foundation of this, but CBT-I also uses cognitive restructuring techniques to change unhelpful thoughts and beliefs about sleep.

(I hope you don't mind, but I have been a little tricksy; I have already been doing that with you. Remember when I asked you to turn your hair blue? Well, there was a reason why I did that and why I made it as absurd as I did. I promise I didn't just do it for my amusement or to piss you off!)

Behavioural intervention

Stimulus control, sleep scheduling and sleep restriction/sleep windows are some of the central and incredibly powerful behavioural components of CBT-I that regulate your sleep drive and break the conditioned response of the bed being a place of wakefulness.

I will talk about these in much greater detail during the remainder of this book.

That, in a nutshell, is CBT-I. But what it is not is therapy!

14

Decisions, Decisions

'Why not?' I thought. 'I have tried everything else, so let's book myself a proper sleep course.' I had seen acupuncturists, reflexologists and a whole host of other 'specialists' in the past –slouching and sloppy or in sequins, dabbling in sleep as a sideshow. I was done with that. This time I wanted a business that specialised in sleep and only sleep.

I scoured the internet and narrowed it down to two possibilities.

Harley Street (very, very posh) in London. On this course, you went into a lab overnight where you would be wired up, and people in white coats with lots of letters after their names would look at screens that go 'bing' and make notes on a clipboard so they knew what was wrong with you and you could see for yourself exactly what was going on with your sleep. (Oh, so it turns out at 3.22 am I thought I was awake, but I was actually asleep; that's interesting, here's £50,000.)

The course I ended up going for was an eight-week CBT-I course. No lab, no white coats and no machine that went 'bing'.

It was a tough decision. 'I have a serious problem with my brain here,' I thought. Surely, I need the machine that goes 'bing'.

But it turns out I didn't. And it also turned out that the choice I made was the most important decision of my life!

Sleep Knowledge 14
Do sleep trackers help you sleep?

Track your run, track your steps, track your heartbeat, track all the minutiae of your entire existence.

Have you tracked your sleep? Does tracking it decrease your anxiety and obsession with sleep? Does having something tell you that (based on the arbitrary rule that we must all get 8 hours' sleep) you slept poorly last night give you better-quality sleep over the long term?

Simply put, do you feel you are sleeping better because you have tracked your sleep or are tracking it now?

And are sleep trackers accurate? The machines they use in sleep labs cost tens of thousands of pounds. What people use to track their sleep at home costs a fraction of this and can also be used to order a pizza and watch celebrities on an island eating things they shouldn't for no reason whatsoever.

Don't get me wrong. Sleep trackers are fantastic for the people that sell them, but do they help you sleep?

15

The First Day of My Sleep Course

It was 2 April 2019, the first day of my CBT-I course. In the morning, I logged onto my computer. A short while later, I was waiting for the first session to begin.

Did I genuinely think that this course would help? No. I wanted it to. I desired that more than anything. But I didn't. I couldn't. All the evidence from the past told me that everything I tried didn't work, so I had no confidence whatsoever that this would be any different.

That changed dramatically within about 5 minutes.

My course started. The person running it was incredibly warm, kind and friendly, so I felt relaxed instantly. Since I still thought CBT-I was therapy (of course – that's what it says it is!), I instantly took on the role of patient and started down that road.

'You see, I'm going through a divorce which I am finding stressful, so I think about that at night … and whenever I feel more stressed, my insomnia seems to be worse. I had acute insomnia during my….'

In the kindest possible way, I was interrupted.

'This isn't counselling,' they said.

That stopped me dead. I was expecting to comb through my past and my current life to find the stressor preventing me from sleeping.

But within 2 minutes, I realised that it wasn't going to happen.

I then went on to talk about the severity of my insomnia. Before the course, I had already filled in a questionnaire littered with my insomnia problems. You know what they are – anxiety, fear, frustration, anger, rituals, pleading, sleeping pills, erratic schedule etc.

I was convinced that my insomnia would be the worst insomnia they had ever seen in their life.

I was also expecting them to have never heard anything like my behaviours ever before. I expected to be validated in my conviction with a comment that ran something like this.

'My goodness, Joseph, I have never seen a case like this; you eat two kiwi fruit, have a hot bath, obsess and worry about sleep, and you sleep late into the day to catch up on it! Your insomnia is documentary bad. I'm going to need to bring in a whole team of scientists to work on this case.'

I didn't get the validation I was expecting. What I got instead was

'That's all incredibly common. Your insomnia is about average.'

That's it! Average. Middle of the road, ordinary, middling, typical, average.

I thought to myself that if my insomnia were a bird, it would be a seagull. They steal your chips, so they can be a bit of nuisance, but other than that, they are pretty unremarkable.

Usually, when you have your colours nailed to the mast and see them come up tattered and faded, that can be a blow to your ego.

But not in this case. Average! Oh, what joy!

I wasn't prepared to give up the fight and hand over all my convictions quite so easily, however.

I was wrong that I would have to unpick the trigger of my insomnia to solve it, and I was wrong about the assumption that my insomnia was unique to me and incredibly severe. But third time's a charm.

'You see, I have found that this relaxation technique can sometimes work, and if I meditate on a Tuesday on the first quarter of the moon cycle then … and did you know that that 5HTP contains serotonin which … And well, you see, erm, gosh.'

None of it worked. I know now that none of what I had tried had worked, and it never had, and deep down, I knew it then as well.

But I had spent so long obsessing, trawling through the articles on the internet, educating myself about sleep. I'd spent hours researching the different chemicals in the brain. I'd tried sleeping late into the morning to catch up, sleeping in different positions, learning every relaxation technique under the sun. Nothing I had done up to that point led to consistent, quality sleep over the long term. None of it, but it is tough to come to terms with the fact that you haven't had a clue what you were doing and have spent twenty years of your life making everything worse.

Twenty years! Twenty years of fighting sleep. Twenty years of anger, stress and torment night after night. I had lost my business, lost my marriage, lost my best friend. My life was in tatters, and it had all been for nothing.

'Oh Mr Pannell,' I thought 'one's been such a silly little goose.'

Now I know I was incredibly hard on myself. But in life, if you act unskilfully or stupidly, it is essential to be critical and talk roughly to yourself as often as possible. Doing so helps to destroy your self-esteem.

While you can often rely on others to do it for you, you really ought to do it yourself if you want something done properly. So I did. And after I had done that, I swept up everything I thought I knew about sleep and dumped it there and then in the bin.

Fair play, I thought. You know how to cure insomnia, and I don't. I am asking for your help, and I am here to learn. If you tell me what I need to know and what I need to do, I will do it.

And I did.

And now I no longer have insomnia!

Sleep Knowledge 15
Pavlovian/classical conditioning

Classical conditioning is learning by association, where two stimuli are linked together to produce a learnt response.

The most well-known example of classical conditioning was Pavlov's experiment with dogs. In this experiment Ivan Pavlov would ring a bell prior to the dog being fed. After a few repetitions, Pavlov observed that the dog would start to salivate every time the bell was rung. This was because the dog had learnt to associate the sound of the bell with the presentation of food.

'But Joseph,' I hear you say, 'I'm not a greyhound. Sure, in college maybe I experimented with a tennis ball a time or two. But I didn't like it. I didn't chew. And I didn't try it again.'

So what's this got to do with my sleep?

Quite a lot actually.

Classical conditioning doesn't just apply to dogs.

Psychologist John Watson proposed that 'the process of classical conditioning (based on Pavlov's observations) was able to explain all aspects of human psychology. Everything from speech to emotional responses was simply patterns of stimulus and response' (McLeod 2018).

If you eat a kiwi fruit (stimulus) before bed and you happen to sleep (response), the brain will learn, through repetition, to associate eating a kiwi fruit with sleep. But the kiwi fruit does not make you sleep. The opposite is also true. If you were to eat a kiwi fruit and have a dreadful night's sleep, the brain would then associate kiwi fruit with wakefulness, and eating kiwi fruits before bed would cause you anxiety and stress.

What about the bed? Do you ever notice that you can be calm and relaxed and sleepy (perhaps you even fall asleep) when you are downstairs on the sofa watching TV, and the second you get into bed you instantly feel hyperaroused?

Why is this? The bed is a cosy, wonderful, relaxing place to be – or at least it was before you had insomnia.

In this example, the bed is the stimulus, and the brain has associated the bed with hyperarousal and wakefulness (the response).

But there is more to it than this. When you go to bed there is also a shift in intent. When downstairs watching TV, you want to stay awake; wakefulness is desirable, so it is not a threat, and because wakefulness is not a threat, you are not hyperaroused.

But as soon as your head hits the pillow, you don't want to be awake; you want to be asleep. The second that being awake becomes something undesirable, that triggers all the anxious, hyperaroused thought patterns associated with the bed because wakefulness is now a threat. You are still sleepy; sleepiness doesn't just disappear, unless you sleep, but now your hyperarousal is masking your drive to sleep.

So, what's to be done? Well, thankfully, in the same way that the brain has used repetition to associate the bed with wakefulness, the brain can also use repetition to associate the bed with sleep.

And I'll be discussing how to do that next!

16

Putting It into Practice

During my first appointment, within the space of an hour, I had learnt more about sleep than I ever had in my entire life. Also, for the first time in my entire life, I had spoken to someone who understood insomnia. Everything. How it makes you think, how it makes you feel, your behaviours and thought patterns – everything.

Because I completely trusted in their knowledge and experience, I also completely trusted that they knew a way out of insomnia.

If this is the first book about sleep like this one you have ever read, perhaps you are thinking along the same lines. (I say perhaps; the truth is I have no idea what you are thinking. I can't even control my own thoughts half the time, so I certainly can't claim to have any authority over yours!)

If that is the case, that's very good! Thinking like this will be very helpful to you. The behaviour changes that help regulate your sleep drive and gradually untangle the anxious and obsessive thought patterns around sleep are incredibly effective.

I don't know how long you have had your insomnia, but when replacing months or years of ingrained old habits, behaviours and thought patterns with new ones (that work!), it can take a while before they feel natural and automatic.

Also, progress is not linear. Overall, you will find that your sleep improves over the long run, but you will have a few setbacks (speed bumps is a better term) along the way. I certainly did!

That said, what I am sharing with you is quantifiably the most effective, evidence-based, long-term cure for insomnia with decades-worth of research behind it. You need sleep, so as long as the behaviour changes are applied, it will work for you over the long term.

Perhaps from what you have already learnt, you have built up enough trust in the sleep knowledge I have shared with you to know with absolute certainty that through thought-pattern and behaviour changes you can overcome your insomnia, just the same as I overcame mine. That belief will help you during the trickier times, but with consistency, you will get there.

Right – let's do this!

For starters, I did five things that worked for me that you can do too.

1) Only use your bedroom for sleep. Sex is OK too, but no taking the laptop into bed for working, no hula hooping, fire breathing or whatever else you used to get up to in there.

2) Only go to bed when you are can't-keep-your-eyes-open sleepy.

3) If you are in bed, not asleep, and you starting to feel anxious and worried about sleep, get up and go into another room and do something that you enjoy until you feel sleepy again.

4) Get up at the same time every day. Get up, get light, get active!

5) Don't nap.

That's it, the only five pieces of advice I needed to follow. Somebody who has never had insomnia may think that five rules like this are too restrictive. However, over my twenty years of insomnia, I had accumulated thousands of rules: I must do this, I must do that, I must only ... Five rules seemed like nothing in comparison.

What's more, they were not forever, and I didn't need to do everything perfectly (I will cover this later in the book).

These five techniques are behavioural. The B part of CBT-I.

Let's examine them and their purpose individually.

1) Only use the bedroom for sleep.

This advice is to condition your brain to associate both the bed and the bedroom as a place of relaxation, restfulness and sleep. Earlier I discussed Pavlovian conditioning. We are using this principle here.

Over the years, you have conditioned your brain to associate not only the bed with wakefulness, you have also conditioned it to associate the bedroom with wakefulness.

This behavioural technique will condition you to do the opposite.

2) Only go to bed when you are can't-keep-your-eyes-open sleepy.

It is impossible to force sleep and to fall asleep when you are not sleepy. Sleep is a drive state. A natural process. By only going to bed when you are sleepy, you will be doing many things.

Firstly, you will be reducing the amount of time spent in bed trying to force sleep and getting anxious and worried about not sleeping in the process.

This anxiety is the hyperaroused fight-or-flight state. In this state, your adrenaline and cortisol increase, as do your body temperature and heart rate – the exact opposite of what you need for sleep!

Secondly, by reducing the amount of time spent in bed, you will be regulating your sleep drive.

Thirdly, by reducing the amount of time spent in bed not sleeping, you are conditioning the brain to associate the bed with sleep rather than wakefulness.

You may have heard the opposite advice before: set a regular bedtime. But since sleep is a natural process, a drive state, why would we be setting our bedtime by our watch rather than how we feel? Am I sleepy? No, so why am I going to bed? Wouldn't I rather be doing something else I find enjoyable, like watching a film, sitting by the fire or reading a book?

'But Joseph, what if I never feel sleepy, or I can't tell the difference between fatigue and sleepiness?'

No problem, I will cover all this later in the book!

3) If you are in bed not asleep and start to feel anxious and worried about sleep, get up and go into another room and do something that you enjoy until you feel sleepy again.

If you are in bed, not asleep, think about how you feel. If you feel relaxed, happy and sleepy, wonderful! If you stay there and allow sleep to come, it will. But if you are starting to feel anxious, worried or angry or are trying to force sleep, go into another room and do something that you enjoy until you feel sleepy again.

In CBT-I this is called stimulus control. My problem with sleep was trouble in falling asleep and spending hours in bed trying to force sleep.

Perhaps your problem is waking in the night and then struggling to fall back to sleep and spending hours trying to force it, or perhaps it is waking up early or having poor, fragmented sleep.

As with all the techniques mentioned here and throughout the book, stimulus control will work for you regardless of what type of insomnia you have.

Stimulus control is another technique used to reduce the amount of time spent in bed, becoming anxious and worried and trying to force sleep.

It conditions the brain to start seeing the bed as a place of sleep rather than of wakefulness (Pavlovian conditioning). It is a psychological step away from trying to sleep because you are doing the exact opposite of making yourself sleep.

By being awake but doing something that you enjoy and that makes you happy, you are also teaching the brain that wakefulness is not something to fear and not something that is a threat.

And when wakefulness stops becoming a threat, you stop fearing it, and when you stop fearing wakefulness, you relax, and you sleep!

4) Get up at the same time every day. Get up. Get light. Get active!

Getting up at the same time every day is one of, if not **the single** most important piece of advice for sleep.

Getting up at the same time everyday anchors your circadian drive for wakefulness and your homoeostatic sleep pressure.

You cannot force sleep in the short term at night, but you can certainly create a strong, regulated sleep drive at the start of your day for good-quality sleep in the long term.

Get light! Lots of it. Natural or artificial, either way, as soon as possible and in the first third of your day, get plenty of light to get yourself all bright-eyed and bushy-tailed. (I'll discuss the importance of light in the next Sleep Knowledge section.)

Get active.

Endorphins. Serotonin. Dopamine. Norepinephrine. They're nice. You want them. They're proper lush. They are also sending alerting signals to the brain at the time you want it to be alert and thereby regulating your sleep drive.

5) Don't nap.

Again, the purpose of this advice is to regulate the sleep drive, letting the body know that to get sleep (which it needs) it had better start giving it to you when you want it. At night.

You have to sit it down and talk firmly to your sleep drive from time to time, or it just runs amok and does whatever it wants.

These, then, were my five pieces of advice. They were the opposite of what I had been doing up to this point. But that's great, right?

Nothing I had done up to this point had worked, so why would I want to do the same things again?

The time I chose to wake up in the morning was 6.30 am. But what if I only felt like I had slept for 2 hours? I'm not going to get up at 6.30 am then am I? Actually yes. That was difficult, saying no to short-term sleep when it was on offer. But I had been snatching short-term sleep whenever I could for twenty years, and had it worked?

Did I want sleep in the short term, or did I want long-term good-quality sleep and to put my insomnia behind me for good?

Sleep Knowledge 16
Light!

Several studies report that daytime exposure to white light enriched in short-wavelength content was associated with increased evening fatigue and sleep quality, decreased sleep-onset latency, and increased slow-wave sleep accumulation. (Blume et al. 2019)

Exposure to bright light as soon as possible and in the first third of your day helps to regulate the hormones that affect wakefulness and sleep drive.

If you can get into the habit of getting as much bright light as you possibly can, as soon as you can, this has been proven to help you fall asleep faster, decrease night-time awakenings, and improve your sleep quality. Fantastic!

As for screens and blue light at night, you can find a link to an article by the University of Manchester in the References section to read more about this, but the evidence that blue light causes insomnia is not only conflicting but has also been completely overblown. For example, one study concluded that people who read from iPads for hours before bed took on average only 10 minutes longer to fall asleep than people who read from a paperback.

10 minutes! That doesn't sound like an insomnia problem to me.

Do normal sleepers not watch films before bed?

And what is avoiding blue light? An avoidance sleep effort, and I'm not taking you down that rabbit hole again. So, if you have a film you want to watch before bed, get stuck in!

17

Come on Eileen – Get Stuck In!

That night and for the next two weeks, I had five, easy to follow, evidence-based steps that had been proven to work in controlled scientific studies with over three decades' worth of data ready to put into action.

When I compared them side by side with the insomnia techniques I had developed myself over the past two decades (JPRT-I ™ Joseph Pannell Ridiculous Techniques for Insomnia), which I had proven with a vast body of evidence most certainly did not work, I had to admit CBT-I was the far superior model.

So I put these steps into practice that night and for the following two weeks, until my next appointment.

So how did I get on? After two weeks, was I sleeping like I used to before I had insomnia?

No. I was still sleeping poorly, but actually, while it didn't feel like it at the time, because the results were not groundbreaking and I didn't feel any better during the day, I had already made significant improvements.

I had better nights, and I had poor nights. Still, overall, my sleep quality and duration had slightly improved.

I was also taking lower doses of my sleeping tablets, and I now had structure to my sleep.

I was going to bed around 11 pm and was awake at 7 am. (I was still trying to force 8 hours of sleep, but undoing twenty years of bad habits wasn't going to happen overnight!)

My anxiety was definitely still there, but what made a huge difference was knowing that I could get out of bed when I wasn't sleeping.

Not only did it feel better to do that in the short term, I also knew it was helpful to my sleep in the long term.

The door had been left wide open, and I could leave my bed any time I wanted. So I did!

Sleep Knowledge 17
Stimulus control

I don't like ironing. I don't like scrolling through my phone. Neither of these are treats to me and something that I enjoy. So I didn't do either of these things during my stimulus control.

I like to sit in front of the fire and read a book; it's what I enjoy. But there is more than one way to massage a moose (I use rollers). So what do you enjoy and would look forward to doing at night-time?

When you are doing your own stimulus control, if you are in bed and you feel relaxed and happy, wonderful! If you stay there and allow sleep to come, it will. But if you feel that anxiety is starting to creep up on you and you feel yourself trying to force sleep, kill the beast when it is little and give yourself permission, instead of worrying, to go and do something that you absolutely love.

Avoid computers and avoid phones; both of these devices the brain can associate with work, worry and wakefulness, and there are too many distractions and rabbit holes to fall down with them. I would also advise against computer games.

Make sure you set up your area before bed to make engaging in that activity as easy as possible. (In my case, book on the coffee table, reading light on!) Only return to bed when you feel sleepy again. Especially during the early stages of stimulus control, you may need to leave the bedroom more than once – or even multiple times during the night.

Does stimulus control work immediately? No. It isn't a secret weapon that guarantees sleep. But little by little, the anxiety associated with not being able to fall asleep will gradually lessen as the brain is conditioned that wakefulness is not a threat (quite the opposite; if you do something you love at night when you are awake, then there is nothing to fear from being awake) and that the bed is a place for sleep!

18

Stimulus Control and Sleep Scheduling as a Path to Normal Sleep

Towards the end of my second week of stimulus control, I was already starting to feel that my anxiety around being in bed was starting to reduce.

'But there is a problem,' I thought to myself. 'This isn't what normal sleepers do is it?'

Are they not just as happy in bed awake as asleep? Yes. Awake, asleep, just happy to be there. A place of 'non-attachment to the outcome' like I have now, and what you used to have before insomnia.

You'll get back there too, and when you do, you won't feel the need to be getting out of bed.

Suppose I use an analogy here. When I first learnt to ride a bike, I had stabilisers. Then, my father held onto the back of my bike and ran alongside me. Then, he let go, and I did great until I cycled into a hedge. My father then went back to holding onto the back of me until he let go again, and I did it all by myself. And as my confidence grew, I got better and better.

But that was last year. Now at only 36 years of age, I have got rid of my old bike with the stabilisers and playing cards in the spokes and replaced it with a mountain bike that I go down hills on and cycle one-handed and everything!

Sleep windows (coming up) and stimulus control are there for you when you need them but only as a tool to help you become a normal sleeper. They are not the end goal. The purpose of them is to help you transition away from them.

For me and for the many people with insomnia who have got used to controlling their sleep (in a way that isn't helpful), going from controlling sleep to nothing is too big a jump. This is where the stimulus-control and sleep-window structure is helpful in the initial stages. Stimulus control and sleep windows are just a stepping stone towards 'normal sleep', and I will talk about normal sleep now!

Sleep Knowledge 18
Normal sleep

I have written a lot about normal sleep and normal sleepers. But what is a 'normal sleeper?' Well, as we know, it is not typical for the average person who sleeps well to get 8 hours of sleep, and actually closer to 6 hours is far more usual.

Also, as we learnt in the Sleep Knowledge section 'The stages of sleep', normal sleepers also wake during the night and spend a proportion of their time during the night in bed awake rather than asleep. It is normal to experience some wakefulness during the night; everybody does!

Furthermore, normal sleepers do not sleep well every night. Typically, they will sleep well 70% of the time.

Normal sleepers will also typically respond to stressful events by sleeping poorly for a period. Imagine if somebody told you that their dog had died last night and they slept like a baby. That would be less normal than sleeping poorly.

A normal sleeper is just somebody who has a healthy relationship with sleep; they don't worry and obsess about sleep, and they don't spend hours in bed trying to force it. Poor sleep, good sleep, no problem – it's all the same to a normal sleeper, and a 'normal sleeper' is what this book is here to help you become!

19

My Second Sleep Appointment

It was 16 April 2019. I had completed the first two weeks of my eight-week sleep course, and I was now sat talking to my sleep specialist again.

I had done it. It had not been easy, but I had done it. Even the part that I found difficult, getting up at the same time every day, I had done. I had chosen the long-term benefits over the short-term instant quick fix for that day. It was hard. It didn't make me feel good, but the prospect of twenty, thirty, forty more years of insomnia felt much worse.

What was also liberating was that I hadn't indulged in any of my normal rituals for two weeks.

Five very clear-cut ones had replaced all my normal rules around how to force sleep.

The improvements were admittedly small, but they were happening.

I should have been happy with the results, but I wasn't. I wasn't, because I still couldn't detect any improvements during the day regarding how I felt. I still felt anxious and irritable; I was still trying to force sleep.

I was also furious with myself when I failed to sleep on any given night in the short term.

When I went downstairs during my stimulus control after I had failed to make myself sleep, I viewed this through the lens of defeat.

I was obsessed with sleep duration and measured my success and improvements in my sleep purely by the amount of time I felt I had slept that night. Tuesday: 3 hours – bad! Friday: 5 hours 34 minutes – good!

Was thinking like this helping me during my course? Not particularly. So, when I spoke to my sleep specialist during my second appointment, how did they help me change how I thought about sleep and how did they help me change how I measured my perception of success? And if you find yourself focusing only on sleep duration and becoming angry or despondent during the nights you don't sleep as well as you would have liked, what would be helpful for you to focus on instead?

Well, firstly, they pointed out that changing my behaviours, especially twenty years of ingrained ones, was hard, and despite that, I was doing it!

When you follow the five steps above and change your own ingrained behaviours, that will be hard too, so the fact you are doing it is fantastic!

Secondly, they showed me that I could have measured my success not on how well I had slept on any given night, or how many times I went downstairs during the night but how I responded to the poor night's sleep or how I responded to going downstairs. Did I respond by giving up and going back to my old behaviours? No, I responded by sticking at it.

Thirdly, I came to see that I could have focused on my successes. I had reduced my sleeping tablets. I had a regular sleep schedule, and despite the speed bumps, there had been a few nights where I had slept reasonably well and woken up early.

On your path towards better sleep, compare yourself to the sleeper you were when you first started, rather than the one you would like to be today.

I had had insomnia for twenty years, so to see small improvements in only two weeks – that's incredible! I should have told everybody about my successes and shouted them from the rooftops, and I would encourage you to do just that!

But what if your sleep doesn't improve in the first couple of weeks? What if it gets worse? Well, that can sometimes happen too; in fact, it is common! What does a toddler do when it wants your attention? It kicks and it screams more and more loudly until it gets it.

Your insomnia can do this too. It says to you, 'Hey! You need to stop doing this; you used to get at least some sleep when you slept late into the morning, so what on earth are you doing? I feel scared and threatened. What you are doing is dangerous; give me some attention!' It kicks and screams and tries to grab as much of your attention as it can, and when it does this, you can sleep worse.

So what do you do if your insomnia gets worse after you first adopt these new behaviour changes? You do exactly what the old-school parents do when their toddler starts having a tantrum: you ignore it. You carry on just as before, and eventually it settles down and starts to play with its toys. (Credit to Martin Reed for this. He refers to this as 'insomnia's extinction burst'. Extinction bursts can also come later during your treatment. You can watch a YouTube video about the extinction burst by following the link to Martin Reed's materials in the Resources section of this book).

Taken as a whole, my insomnia didn't have an extinction burst. Some nights it did; there were a few nights in a row I slept worse than I had in years, but, overall in the two-week period, I slept slightly better than I had been. I should have celebrated every one of my successes. But that wasn't how I reacted. I didn't react like this, because I wanted instant results. Of course, I wanted instant results. I had lived with insomnia for twenty years, and I wanted to be rid of it.

That's why supplements, relaxation techniques, kiwi fruit and sleeping pills are so alluring. They offer the promise of instant results, but that is all it is – a promise, a promise that is never delivered.

Overcoming insomnia isn't about instant results. It's about consistency.

'We are what we repeatedly do.' (Will Durant)

And two weeks? Well, that's not repeatedly. I had built my insomnia brick by brick for twenty years, to dismantle everything in fourteen days – come now, Mr Pannell, be realistic!

But still. I wanted something dramatic. Thankfully, I was going to get it!

Looking back at the first two weeks of my five new behaviour changes, there was a habit I hadn't quite got to: 'Only go to bed when you are sleepy.'

I was consistently going to bed around 11 pm and getting up at 7 am. That's 8 hours in bed. The time we are told we all need.

But was I going to bed when I was sleepy? No. And the reason was that I still didn't know what actual sleepiness was.

So the next step of the course was to give me an awareness of what sleepiness was and to get long periods of good-quality sleep ingrained into my system again.

To do this, I was going to give my body less of an opportunity to sleep by reducing the amount of time spent in bed. (Sounds lovely, right? I don't anymore, but I still saw the bed as a place of stress and anxiety. Spending less time in it! Fantastic!)

And for this I had a sleep window to stick to. (I will show you how to do your own sleep window very soon.)

With my new sleep window set, despite the fact that I was look-ing forward to spending less time in bed and more time doing the things I loved, I was still a little apprehensive.

During my insomnia, I read countless articles on the internet and in newspapers telling me in no uncertain terms that we must get 8 hours of sleep and that sleep deprivation causes a whole host of health problems.

And there I was on a sleep programme that was going to restrict my time in bed in the short term, to help me sleep in the long term. I was worried about that, but should I have been con-cerned? Well, the next Sleep Knowledge section will help an-swer that question!

Sleep Knowledge 19
Correlation is not causation

Sleep windows are put in place to limit the amount of time spent in bed which **may** result in a shorter sleep duration in the short term. (I say 'may' as when using my own sleep window, despite spending less time in bed, I actually slept a lot more because I spent the vast majority of my time in bed actually asleep!)

Some people who do not have sleep problems may just be 'short sleepers' and typically sleep for less than 6 hours but don't want or need any more sleep.

That is until they open up a newspaper or click on a website article that tells them that their feet will explode if they don't get 8 hours of sleep. They were fine before, but now, all of a sudden, they are worried they will burst into flames if they don't get the recommended amount of sleep.

To help put your mind at rest about the perceived dangers of 'short sleep' (sleeping for less than 6 hours) and also deliberately choosing to restrict your time in bed using a sleep window, I'm going to use an analogy from my tutor Daniel Erichsen.

Did you know that there is a strong correlation between ashtrays and COPD (chronic obstructive pulmonary disease)?

Not only is there a strong correlation between the two, but there is also a dose-response relationship. The more ashtrays people have, the greater the likelihood of lung problems.

That's bad. Ashtrays are therefore incredibly dangerous.

But do ashtrays cause COPD or is it smoking that causes COPD? Of course, it is smokers who also tend to have ashtrays.

The above example shows a correlation between COPD and ashtrays, but ashtrays are not what causes COPD.

What has this got to do with 'short sleep' and health concerns?

Everything! There are correlations between short sleep and certain health concerns, but short sleep has never been proven to cause health concerns.

120

Let's look first at the feasibility of proving that short sleep causes, for example, Alzheimer's disease. To prove that one thing causes another, you will need a randomized study with two imposed conditions. You need thousands of people, and you need to make half of them sleep-deprived as you make sure the other half sleep a lot. After decades of maintaining both groups of short and long sleepers, respectively, you could look at whether Alzheimer's happened more in the sleep deprived or non sleep deprived group (Erichsen 2019).

What's the likelihood of that study ever happening? Even if it were financially viable and possible to conduct (which it isn't), if you were a normal sleeper, would you sign up for this study?

So why does a correlation even exist between short sleep and health concerns?

As discussed earlier in the Sleep Knowledge section, 'The stages of sleep', certain health concerns can mean you wake more frequently during the night or become more aware of waking in the night.

Let's take fibromyalgia as an example.

Suppose you wake more frequently due to fibromyalgia and lack understanding of how to prevent this from turning into a sleep problem. In this case, you may start to become anxious about not sleeping, develop a sleep problem in consequence and end up sleeping less.

A correlation has now been found between fibromyalgia and 'short sleep'. But the 'short sleep' did not cause fibromyalgia.

Also, somebody with fibromyalgia who does not have a sleep problem may, due to their condition, be more aware of waking often in the night than somebody who does not have that health concern. But in reality, the person isn't sleeping any less; they are just reporting their sleep duration more accurately.

But again, a correlation has been found between 'short sleep' and fibromyalgia.

But the opposite is also true. People with fibromyalgia can also feel fatigued, which can cause them to spend more time in bed than average. Because they spend more time in bed, they may also report that they sleep for over 8 hours a night on average.

They may well sleep for over 8 hours a night, or they may just be overestimating how long they sleep – either way, a correlation has been found between fibromyalgia and sleeping for over 8 hours.

A whole host of health concerns can result in people spending longer in bed and overestimating the amount of time they sleep, so the correlation between health concerns and sleeping for over 8 hours is actually more substantial than the link between health concerns and sleeping for less than 6 hours.

But this is often conveniently overlooked.

If you were a normal sleeper who sleeps for 6 hours a night on average, would you buy a new mattress, a weighted blanket, a supplement, a grounding sheet, click on that article or pick up that newspaper in an attempt to increase the amount of time you slept if you read that long sleeping was linked to a whole host of health concerns?

Probably not.

So, don't panic! I had a sleep window and didn't spontaneously combust, and nor you will you. What you will do, however, is sleep!

20

The World's Shortest, Most Irrelevant Chapter, so I Can Shoehorn in a Sleep Knowledge Section

I don't watch a lot of TV. But you know what I like? *The Great British Bake Off.* There is no nastiness. It's just lovely people making lovely cakes in a tent and Prue complaining about things that are meant to be incredibly sweet being too sweet.

That and old episodes of *The Crystal Maze* with Richard O'Brien

Sleep Knowledge 20
Sleep windows

To sleep more and to get better quality sleep, you should spend less time in bed.

Important: This book is to provide sleep knowledge. It is not here to tell you do anything. You have a legal obligation not to drive or operate heavy machinery if you are feeling sleepy.

I had been spending 9, 10, 11, 12 hours in bed. But how much was I sleeping, and what good had it been doing me?

None. The longer I spent there, the more it fed my anxiety and the less I slept.

How long do you spend in bed, and how long do you feel you are actually sleeping? Is that helping you?

Perhaps like me, your sleep schedule was (or is) so erratic that you may not know how long you spend in bed or how long you spend asleep as that changes all the time.

But very roughly, how long do you feel you are sleeping?

You may say that you feel you are only sleeping 2 to 3 hours a night but spending 9 hours in bed (this is how I have felt in the past, but you will be sleeping longer).

Nine hours in bed, but you feel you are only sleeping for two or three of them? That's a lot of time that you could be using to do something you enjoy.

Now you know that less time in bed leads to longer and better-quality sleep. Perhaps you might think about how long you would like to spend in bed and what would be realistic.

Go a bit Goldilocks and the three bears, when trying to come up with the answer.

8 hours – too soft! The average time a normal sleeper sleeps is a bit above 6 hours. Do you need to spend 8 hours in bed?

4 hours – too hard! You should always give yourself a good opportunity to sleep, and it should never be below 5 hours. Remember, even if you think you are only sleeping 2–3 hours,

you will be sleeping more. It will just be very fragmented and poor-quality sleep that you are getting.

5.5–6.5 hours (possibly 7 at the upper end) – just right! 5.5 hours is less than the average time normal sleepers sleep, so it is a little on the extreme side and being a bit rough on yourself. 6 to 6.5, maybe? It's up to you.

If, for example, you have chosen 6 hours to be in bed, set your morning time to whenever you want. Let us say 6.30 am, so you should make sure you go to bed after 12.30 am. That doesn't mean you must go to bed at 12.30 am as you still should only go to bed when you feel sleepy. But try to make sure that it is after 12.30 am.

This 6 hour sleep window isn't forever. When you start feeling that you are falling asleep more quickly or waking up less frequently or still waking up in the night (which is what normal sleepers do) but falling back to sleep faster, in short, when you feel your sleep quality is improving and you would like to, perhaps extend the time you have in bed by 15 minutes or so every week.

Does it have to be 15 minutes, and does it have to be every week? No. Try not to do it too quickly, but it's your sleep, so it's your decision. You understand how sleep works now, so trust yourself to make the right one!

After a month, six weeks or perhaps two months, you will eventually reach a point where you no longer feel you would like more time in bed. Wonderful!

You now know how long you personally like to spend in bed to get good-quality sleep.

Once you know your new sleep window, does that mean you now have to have that sleep window for the rest of your life?

No. Normal sleepers don't have such rigid time frames. They have a healthy relationship with sleep. They go to bed when they are sleepy and get up at the same time most days. And normal sleep is what you will have!

How did I get on with my own sleep window? Well you're about to find out.

21

Steamy Sleep Drives

I had completed the first two weeks of my course. I was now on weeks 2–4 and on the first night of my sleep window. That night I made sure I went to bed after my allotted time, excited to see the results and expecting to fall asleep a little bit quicker. And what happened? Nothing.

I had a poor night's sleep of only a few hours. But hey ho, I was doing it!

On my second night again, I went to bed after my allotted time and again. Nothing. A reasonable sleep but no better than I had been getting.

The third. Nothing.

The fourth. Better but not great. But I kept at it.

The fifth – now the fifth was different. Very, very different. Oh, my giddy aunt, it was what-on-earth-is-happening-to-me different!

It was 10 pm or so when sleepiness started to build. I still hadn't truly known what sleepiness was up to that point, but my Goodness, I was about to find out.

My eyelids were starting to droop and get heavy. The stress and anxiety that I usually feel before going to bed was replaced with a calming anaesthesia.

Yawns were coming thick and fast, and at 11 pm when I took the dog out for her night-time wee, I was staggering around like I'd just polished off an entire bottle of Christmas home-made moonshine.

Back in the house, I looked at the clock: 11.05. I still had ages until I could go to bed. How on earth was I going to stay awake, I thought.

I started walking in circles around the living room. I stood up against the wall and, just for a second, shut my eyes; it was then I found myself starting to slowly slide down it as I drifted off to sleep.

Into the bathroom I went, where I splashed my face with cold water, pinched my arm, tweaked my earlobe, pushed my eyelids open and fought with everything I had to stay awake.

When my sleep window started, I staggered upstairs. None of the usual anxiety or stress accompanied my usual ascent to the bedroom, not a bit of it.

The bed was there, and I could't wait to get into it. I fell in, fully clothed, and that was it. Gone.

We had been apart for twenty years, but on 21 April 2019 my sleep drive came back.

Abruptly and definitely.

It didn't ask if we could meet to talk about my behaviours that had caused it to leave in the first place, sit me down in a nice tearoom and say,

'I never knew where I stood with you, Joseph, you were always so inconsistent.'

'Yes, yes, I know. I'm sorry. If I can explain, you see ...'

'And another thing. What was it with always cancelling all the fun things we had planned last minute and replacing them with yet another hot bath? Boring! It's like you read that book by that guy with the nice haircut and admittedly impressive cheek-bones and went all weird and overprotective on me, and I never felt understood again.'

That didn't happen.

There was no tearoom and polite conversation. My sleep drive didn't ask if we could take it slow because it was still a little uncertain. No, no, no. None of that.

What did happen is that it snuck into the house, put on a big pair of steel-toe-capped boots, kicked the bedroom door off the hinges, leapt under the covers and started nibbling on my ear-lobe.

Quite frankly, it was too much.

It was an astounding thing to happen. I had spent twenty years doing everything I could to try and force myself to sleep. But within five days of starting my sleep window, I was doing everything I could to force myself to stay awake. And I was failing. Miserably.

Over the next couple of weeks, I tried everything I could to stay awake in the evenings. Sitting on the sofa, I would choose the most adrenaline-inducing action film I could find. I'd close my eyes momentarily, and then wake up with pins and needles in my legs to find the film had finished half an hour ago.

I read books, listened to engaging podcasts and generally did everything in my power to keep my eyes open, but most nights I would fall fast sleep on the sofa; that hadn't happened to me in years, but now it was a regular occurrence.

One night I took to pounding the streets, pleading for rain, in the vain hope it would keep me more alert. I would longingly eye up park benches but be too afraid to sit on them.

What would happen if my sleep drive snuck up behind me? I thought. I'd almost certainly have to deal with the village gossip if, looking slightly dishevelled, Betty caught me walking home at 6 am when she went to pick up her morning paper.

I was over the moon with the results I was getting.

I was sleeping better than I had for years. By the end of the second week, I increased my time in bed and was already sleeping longer, more consistently and with far better quality.

But is restricting sleep normal sleep? No. But that was to come.

Sleep Knowledge 21
Sleep windows as a path to normal sleep

At university, after I had put a joke in my academic essay for the second time running, my favourite tutor pulled me aside and said to me,

'Joseph, I know you're not going to listen to me – I didn't listen either when I was given the same advice, and I'm glad I didn't – but the world will do its best to knock the corners off you, and you will find it an awful lot easier to navigate if you can at least make some effort to pretend that it has.'

So, if you are of a gentle disposition and were not expecting the phrase 'nibbling on my ear lobe' in a book about insomnia, I can only apologise. My tutor was right. I didn't listen.

I am going to repeat four fundamental points about sleep below.

1) Our behaviours perpetuate our insomnia.
2) Sleep is a drive state.
3) Insomnia is not the same as sleep deprivation.
4) There is nothing you can do to force sleep if you are not already sleepy.

These four fundamental points are 100% true and have been proven on countless occasions during randomised trials. But do you wholeheartedly 100% believe them? Perhaps the answer is no. I was the same until I put a sleep window in place, and after I had, there was no question, no doubt in my mind that they were true.

It was fun to describe my sleep drive the way I did, but it hadn't vanished for twenty years in reality. Every single time I had slept, it was because I had a drive to sleep.

What was different, however, was that my sleep drive was now regulated. I had also made my sleep drive so strong that even if there was still some hyperarousal, my sleep drive cut right through it, and I slept anyway.

But normal sleepers don't need to restrict their sleep in order to become so sleepy they physically can't keep their eyes open, do they?

No.

For me, the main reason why my sleep window was so effective wasn't because it made me so sleepy that it overrode my anxiety. No. The main thing it did for me was to give me a psychological leap.

It gave me a sense of certainty.

Proving to myself so dramatically that there was nothing wrong with me or with my ability to sleep gave me the confidence to let go of all the other behaviours I had been using to try to force sleep; it shifted my confidence back to me and my innate ability to sleep.

I know for absolute certain I can sleep, I told myself. And once you start to trust wholeheartedly that sleep is a natural process, a drive state, that you don't have to do anything to force or cajole it and that it will come anyway, then your anxiety around sleep virtually vanishes.

By actively choosing to spend less time in bed and doing the opposite of what your brain is telling you to do, you are also teaching and conditioning your brain that sleeping less is not a threat, only a perceived threat. And what happens when sleeping less stops becoming a threat? You sleep more!

Overcoming insomnia is a path to less effort and eventually no effort to sleep.

Sleep windows are a fundamental step on that path that help you get to a 'no effort' destination. But they are just a tool that is there to be let go of when you no longer need it.

Ask a normal sleeper what they do to sleep well, and they will all tell you the same thing: 'Nothing'.

And now that we have covered sleep windows, for the remainder of the book, I will be teaching you to do nothing.

22

Third Session: Mistakes or Opportunities?

It was now 30 April 2019 I was on the third session of my course. One month in, and I had finished the second week of my sleep window. I was buzzing. Admittedly, some nights during the sleep window, I still slept poorly, but, overall, the vast majority of my time in bed was spent asleep rather than awake, which was such a relief.

I was sleeping so well I had also had the confidence to add more time to my sleep window.

I've cracked it I, thought. As long as I always restrict my sleep and always control my sleep by using a sleep window, then I will be able to sleep.

I hadn't resolved my insomnia, admittedly, but I had come to some truce with it ('OK insomnia, I will promise to stop doing this, this and this, and I promise always to do this, this and this if you promise not to be as unkind to me as you used to be? Deal?')

But wasn't that just more rules and restrictions? Yes. And was I now a normal sleeper? No, but I was getting there.

The sleep window had been fantastic at reducing my anxiety by giving me the certainty that I could sleep, but there was still definitely some apprehension remaining. That wasn't surprising. I had been anxious about sleep for twenty years, so expecting it to vanish entirely after one month was a big ask. But I had definitely made huge improvements.

As well as anxiety when in bed, I still felt some anxiety start to build as bedtime approached. So, what was to be done? Well, the next piece of sleep knowledge that my sleep specialist taught me (among many other things) during my third session will provide you with a technique that will help you feel more grounded in the evenings before bed and take away some of those anxious thoughts. It worked wonders for me, and I am sure it will be just as effective for you.

Sleep Knowledge 22
The buffer zone

If you are currently working with a sleep window, you can use the buffer zone before that sleep window starts.

Say your sleep window starts at 12 am, at 10 pm, 10.30 pm or 11 pm, depending on how much time you would like to give yourself – 1–2 hours is great – make sure all your work is done (you've taken the dog out, done the washing up, locked the house etc.), so you are free to do things you find relaxing and enjoyable. It doesn't matter what they are. Pour yourself a herbal tea, grab a book, put a podcast on. It really doesn't matter. This time is for you, and you can do what you want with it.

This isn't a time to run through a list of relaxation techniques in order to force sleep. If you do anything with the intention of trying to make sleep happen, it is counterproductive. Also, the buffer zone isn't there for you to try to protect sleep. If you fancy going out for a meal, an exercise class or a trip down the pub to hear some music and can't do the buffer zone, no problem!

The purpose of the buffer zone is to train your brain that the time before bedtime is not a threat. Far from it! Setting aside a time when you only do the things that you enjoy will condition your brain to believe that bedtime is something to start looking forward to. And, with consistency, it will!

23

Weeks 4–6 of My Course

Everything was going really well. Not only was I sleeping better, but, after a month of using a sleep window, I was also starting to feel more alert during the day.

When I first started my sleep window, I noticed that even though I was sleeping more, I felt considerably more sleepy during the day compared to when I had insomnia.

You will probably notice this too. Fantastic! Daytime sleepiness is a very good sign that everything you are doing is working for you.

You are getting better-quality sleep. But the reason you feel you are sleepier during the day compared to when you were sleeping less is due to a reduction in hyperarousal.

Hyperarousal doesn't just happen at bedtime. It can occur throughout the day, and by sleeping better and becoming more relaxed and less anxious about sleep, you will start to feel less anxious and more relaxed in general throughout the day. This will also make you feel more sleepy. This is great!

Remember the time before you took action to improve your sleep when you never felt sleepy? Now you are getting that sleepy feeling in spades, and it is a really good thing and a very promising sign.

Day time sleepiness can, however, be a little problematic when you need to get stuff done. Exercise, a nice cup of tea or dancing to your favourite music are all great ways to avoid that nap, so you can get that wonderful, regulated sleep that you want at night-time.

I was sleeping so much better, and I was now feeling more energised during the day.

I was sleeping better because I had followed all the rules and stuck to my sleep window absolutely perfectly.

Or had I?

The wake time I had set during my sleep window was 6.30 am.

Three weeks and five days into my sleep window, I had had a night out on the town for a friend's leaving do.

We weren't just out. We were out out. Restaurant, pubs, clubs, traffic cones on heads. 3 am is when we returned home.

Did I wake up at my new set time of 6.30 am? Not even close. The following morning, I had slept late, very late; I had woken up at 11 am. Over four hours off what it should have been. I had slept late into the morning to catch up on sleep, just like I used to do.

Had I learnt nothing? I was a terrible failure – the worst sleep-course participant in the whole of Devon. I had put all that effort in, and now I had completely wasted it.

It was now 14 May 2019, and I was back on the final session of my sleep course and speaking to my sleep specialist. I thought I'd better come clean, so I confessed to my dreadful indiscretion from two days ago, but not before arming myself for battle by thinking up a whole host of mitigating circumstances to justify my appalling behaviour. In quick succession, I spewed out my excuses.

'Oh, now you see, it was a leaving do. She was going away for a while. We went out to a night club. I didn't want to go ...'

I was stopped halfway through my diatribe. 'That sounds lovely,' they said. 'Was it fun?'

As soon as they said this, I learnt something hugely beneficial that really helped me. I am sure it will help you too. To overcome your insomnia and change your behaviours and thought patterns around sleep, you don't need to be perfect. You just need to be

Good enough.

That's all.

CBT-I isn't about doing something perfectly or really well once and then your sleep will be fixed. It is about changing your relationship with sleep over the long term through repetition and habit building. And for new habits to form, you don't need to do your new behaviours perfectly all the time. You just need to do them more often than not. That's all.

The purpose of everything that I was taught and that I am now sharing with you is to have a healthy relationship with sleep in order to become a 'normal sleeper'.

Normal sleepers don't do everything perfectly all the time. So if 'normal sleep' is perfect sleep, you need to do things 'imperfectly'.

Get up late one day during your sleep window. Well done! Normal sleepers have lie-ins and they still sleep fine. Getting up late during your sleep window will help you transition much more easily to 'normal sleep', so getting up late during your sleep window – genius! What a sage thing for you to have done!

Go to bed early while on your sleep window because you can't keep your eyes open. Wonderful! That just shows how your sleep widow is working for you and that your anxiety has reduced to such a low level that you now really look forward to bed. That's excellent news.

Changing thought processes and behaviours built up over many years can be a little tricky at times, so a little self-compassion and letting go of the need for perfection will help you.

But if that is as unnatural to you as it is to me, the following story from Ajahn Brahm should help.

Ajahn Brahm is a Buddhist monk who moved to Australia after completing a PHD in Astrophysics at the University of Oxford.

He became a monk and, among many other things, set up a monastery in Serpentine, Western Australia. Ajahn Brahm swears and tells toilet jokes. His videos have millions of views, and you can find him on YouTube.

So, if a potty-mouthed British Buddhist sounds like your kind of thing, you're in luck. I present to you a monk on a squashy cushion as a gift (don't unwrap him, it's against his precepts).

Ajahn Brahm teaches through stories. 'Two Bad Bricks in the Wall' is one of my favourites. You can find it in *Opening the Door of Your Heart*.

I met Ajahn Brahm when he visited Gaia House in Devon, and I asked if I could use this story in my book. With his permission, I enclose it in full in the next sleep section.

Sleep Knowledge 23
You don't need to be perfect, just good enough

Two Bad Bricks in the Wall

After we purchased the land for our monastery in 1983 we were broke. We were in debt. There were no buildings on the land, not even a shed. Those first few weeks we slept not on beds but on old doors we had bought cheaply from the salvage yard; we raised them on bricks at each corner to lift them off the ground. (There were no mattresses, of course – we were forest monks.)

The abbot had the best door, the flat one. My door was ribbed with a sizeable hole in the centre where the doorknob would have been. I joked that now I wouldn't need to get out of bed to go to the toilet! The cold truth was, however, that the wind would come up through that hole. I didn't sleep much those nights.

We were poor monks who needed buildings. We couldn't afford to employ a builder – the materials were expensive enough. So I had to learn how to build: how to prepare the foundations, lay concrete and bricks, erect the roof, put in the plumbing – the whole lot. I had been a theoretical physicist and high-school teacher in lay life, not used to working with my hands. After a few years, I became quite skilled at building, even calling my crew the BBC ('Buddhist Building Company'). But when I started it was very difficult.

It may look easy to lay a brick: a dollop of mortar underneath, a little tap here, a little tap there. But when I began laying bricks, I'd tap one corner down to make it level and another corner would go up. So I'd tap that corner down then the brick would move out of line. After I'd nudged it back into line, the first corner would be too high again. Hey, you try it!

Being a monk, I had patience and as much time as I needed. I made sure every single brick was perfect, no matter how long it took. Eventually, I completed my first brick wall and stood back to admire it. It was only then that I noticed – *oh no!* – I'd missed two bricks. All the other bricks were nicely in line, but these two were inclined at an angle. They looked terrible. They spoiled the whole wall. They ruined it.

By then, the cement mortar was too hard for the bricks to be taken out, so I asked the abbot if I could knock the wall down and start over again – or, even better, perhaps blow it up. I'd made a mess of it and I was very embarrassed. The abbot said no, the wall had to stay.

When I showed our first visitors around our fledgling monastery, I always tried to avoid taking them past my brick wall. I hated anyone seeing it. Then one day, some three or four months after I finished it, I was walking with a visitor and he saw the wall.

'That's a nice wall,' he casually remarked.

'Sir,' I replied in surprise, 'have you left your glasses in your car? Are you visually impaired? Can't you see those *two bad bricks* which spoil the whole wall?'

What he said next changed my whole view of that wall, of myself, and of many other aspects of life. He said, 'Yes. I can see those two bad bricks. But I can see the 998 good bricks as well.'

I was stunned. For the first time in over three months, I could see other bricks in that wall apart from the two mistakes. Above, below, to the left and to the right of the bad bricks were good bricks, perfect bricks. Moreover, the perfect bricks were many, many more than the two bad bricks. Before, my eyes would focus exclusively on my two mistakes; I was blind to everything else. That was why I couldn't bear looking at that wall, or having others see it. That was why I wanted to destroy it. Now that I could see the good bricks, the wall didn't look so bad after all. It was, as the visitor had said, 'a nice brick wall.' It's still there now, twenty years later, but I've forgotten exactly where those bad bricks are. I literally cannot see those mistakes anymore.

...

> I have told this anecdote many times. After one occasion, a builder came up to me and told me a professional secret. 'We builders always make mistakes,' he said, 'But we tell our clients that it is "an original feature" with no other house in the neighbourhood like it. And then we charge them a couple of thousand dollars extra!' (Brahm 2015)

We are told we must learn from our failures. And in doing so, if you are anything like me, you will criticise and condemn yourself for them.

But I would hazard a guess you do this far more often to yourself than to others. And will self-criticism and condemnation be helpful to you when overcoming insomnia, or will it just lead to guilt and a loss of confidence in your ability to keep going?

I will put my hands up. Over my twenty years of insomnia, I acted in ways that I wish I hadn't, that were just as hurtful to me as they were to those around me. There were times insomnia got so hard that I isolated myself from my wife and didn't show up for my friends, my family or myself. I stopped living with purpose and became somebody I wouldn't have chosen to be. Slowly but surely, everything I did to try and escape insomnia chipped away at my self-esteem and made me feel that I wasn't good enough and that maybe, if I was honest with myself, there was a small part of me that felt I didn't deserve to be free of it. The erosion of self is a huge component of insomnia, especially if you have lived with it for a long time.

But everything I did – that wasn't me. That was me with insomnia. That was me dealing every day with something I didn't have any control over, that I didn't want and wouldn't have wished on anybody. I didn't understand insomnia, so the actions I took to try and rid myself of it were the best and only things I could do at that time. Nobody can say I didn't try!

Perhaps if you have had insomnia for a long time and have tried to escape it in the same way as I did, you will have done things (or neglected to do things) that were not you, that have chipped away at your self-esteem and made you feel as though you are not good enough; perhaps, like me, there is a small part of you that doesn't feel you deserve to be free of insomnia.

I may be wrong, I frequently am, so whilst that was the case for me, it may well not be the case for you.

But if it is, that isn't or wasn't you. I don't know you, but it doesn't matter, because I know that – like me – you did the best you could. That was then. This is now. You are good enough. You are more than good enough. These behaviour changes can be hard in the short term, but one of the kindest things you can do for yourself is to give yourself the gift of doing them anyway because you know with certainty that you do deserve to overcome your insomnia in the long term. It's time to build a new wall …

Focus on your successes, and, as long as you still have a beautiful wall, you can have as many feature bricks as you want. Normal sleepers do. Normal sleepers also still get poor nights of sleep. Sometimes very poor nights of sleep.

And what do they do about it? Luckily, that was what I would learn in my last session.

24

Finishing Up

I had finished the fourth and final session of my sleep course. During my eight weeks, I had learnt that there was nothing I could do in the short term to force sleep and that anything I did do only fuelled my anxiety and obsession.

I had learnt about avoidance sleep efforts. I had learnt about the homoeostatic sleep drive and the circadian rhythm. And I had learnt how only going to bed when you are sleepy, waking up at the same time every day and spending less time in bed not only strengthens your drive to sleep but also tackles the anxious thoughts surrounding sleep.

I used stimulus control to condition my mind to see the bed as a place of sleep rather than wakefulness and used powerful techniques to massively reduce the hyperarousal that I usually had before bedtime.

This was all wonderful. I used to think that my life circumstances were the only factors that were controlling my sleep. And yet, I was going through a divorce, I had a crumbling business, and I was worried about how I was going to pay the mortgage. My life had fallen on its face. But it didn't matter. None of it. Because I was sleeping – better than I had for twenty years.

Or I was, until one Thursday night four days after my course had ended.

One hour. Two maybe, at most.

Despite everything, all my new behaviour changes, my sleep window, my change in thought patterns, all the sleep knowledge I had learnt and everything I had gone through on my eight-week course, that Friday morning, I woke up at 6.30 am appalled and angry with myself. 'This is how I used to sleep,' I said to myself. 'What has happened?'

I reflected on my night, and as soon as I did, all the anxious, gnawing, stressed thoughts that I used to have came flooding straight back. I had put all that effort into the course, I had tried so hard, but last night I felt like I went straight back to square one.

What had I done? Why had this happened?

That night was horrible. Not just the night itself. I had had many a night like that. That night was dreadful because of the meaning that I gave to it. I had put all that work in, all that effort, and just when I had completed the course and finally felt like I had a handle on insomnia, it blindsides me and kicks me in the teeth. It just seemed so unfair.

But was it unfair? Normal sleepers get bad nights of sleep too. Sometimes they get terrible nights of sleep. But they don't have insomnia.

I had been sleeping amazingly. Just because I had had a bad night of sleep, did that mean that I now had insomnia? No. I had had a bad night of sleep. That's all – nothing else.

'Nothing in life has any meaning except the meaning we give it.' (Robbins 2003, p. 103)

But what if the same thing happens to you? What can you do to fix a bad night's sleep and prevent it from ever happening again? Fortunately, the answer to that question is what I learnt in the fourth session of my course. I'm going to share with you what I learnt by giving you a step-by-step guide now!

Step 1

Instead of sticking to the new behaviours that have given you improved sleep (getting up at the same time, getting light, getting active), you must instead do the opposite.

Lie in bed awake with the curtains drawn and use that opportunity to obsess about the cause. Something like this should do it:

'Hmm, I was told I shouldn't go to bed if I wasn't sleepy, but perhaps I was sleepy, but not sleepy enough and that caused it.'

or

'I shouldn't have watched that television programme as it was a little too stimulating for just before bed. That was a stupid thing to do. Oh, and I had that cup of tea at 3.17 pm when usually I stop drinking caffeine at 3 pm. That probably added to it as well. Oh no! I'm such an idiot. I always do things like this.'

Perfect! You have just inadvertently stumbled onto

Step 2

Berate yourself generally.

This step is critical. You must not skip it. If you don't have to get up, continue with Step 1 and berate yourself in bed.

Lie there for hours to give it the full attention it deserves. If you have to get up, an excellent time to complete this thought is when you are waiting for the kettle to boil.

When you berate yourself generally, be as creative as possible, so it hits home. Make sure you use absolute words like never and always, as these words are fantastic for cognitive distortion. I'll start you off:

'Goodness, Mr Pannell, this kitchen's a mess. When did you last clean out the vegetable drawer? You always do this, and you always will. You will never be any different. Much more of this, and you'll have to apply for meals on wheels.'

'And another thing. Your dog looks like a Jackson Pollock painting. Who can take a man seriously with a dog like that?'

'And while I'm on it – your hair. You used to have such lustrous blonde locks. Now you look like Phil Mitchell. I bet if you oiled your head, small woodland critters would use it as a slippy slide.'

I'm sure you have your own technique. But something along those lines is about right.

Step 3

If not at work, or you don't have to get up, continue with Step 1. If at work, repeatedly tell your work colleagues about how badly you slept just to remind yourself. Most people have at least one person they work with they don't like. For an added bonus, follow them into the toilet, block the door so they can't escape and tell them! They deserve it.

Step 4

This is crucial. You must not, at any point, smile. Remember you didn't sleep as well as you would have liked the previous night, so you must be anxious and stressed and miserable all day. If you start smiling, you're going to tit it right up, so be very careful.

Step 5

When you return home, if you had plans with friends for a fun sporting activity that you enjoy, you must cancel it and instead watch TV (preferably something uneventful that you immediately forget – ITV2 is perfect for this purpose). And while you are watching, quaff a ready meal because you are too emotionally drained to eat properly.

Step 6

Go to bed early to catch up on sleep even if you're not sleepy. Lie there more miserable and fed up with life than you have ever been and do not sleep for a second night.

When you see it on paper, it sounds ridiculous. But I did this. Even two years on from my insomnia, I still do this a little bit. And if you're completely honest, you probably do this, at least to some extent too.

Perfection doesn't exist, nor should it be aimed for. But even if you were to follow your sleep course absolutely perfectly, you will still get bad nights' sleep during your sleep course, and you will still get bad nights' sleep after you have completed it.

'Normal sleepers' sleep well roughly 70% of the time, so even people who have never had insomnia cannot avoid poor nights of sleep. (In fact, there is a significant body of evidence to say that poor nights of sleep are beneficial because they help strengthen the sleep drive. So they are there to help you. But only if you let them!)

Nor can 'normal sleepers' avoid short, stressful situations which may cause a short-term sleep problem.

But they can avoid developing insomnia by following this tip:

'When there is nothing to do, you do nothing slowly and intently' (**Murakami 2002**).

I was taught multiple cognitive restructuring techniques to change my mindset about poor nights' sleep on my sleep course. These were all incredibly helpful, but just knowing you will still get them and don't need to fear them is probably the most important thing to really understand and fully take on board.

From the lofty height of being free from insomnia, it is perhaps easier for me to say 'do nothing' now than it was back then. People generally like to take action to fix problems, so here in the next Sleep Knowledge section are some actual steps you can take.

Sleep Knowledge 24
Responding to a poor night's sleep

After you wake up after a poor night's sleep, say to yourself, 'I would rather have had a good night's sleep, but I will do everything I can to have a great day.'

Get up, get light, get active. Nobody regrets a run after they have done it, and the best and fastest way to feel good again after a poor night's sleep is to do something physical you enjoy.

During the day, get plenty of light. Eat well, and instead of cancelling the things you love, why not reward yourself for not sleeping by doing more of them!

Suppose you do all of this – how well do you think you will sleep the next night?

If you know you can still have a great day after a poor night of sleep, does this diminish the worry about not sleeping?

Training your brain that you can have a poor night's sleep and still have an amazing day is a fantastic way to condition it to recognise that a poor night's sleep is not a threat and not something to fear. Is that something that will benefit your long-term sleep? Oh yes!

Once you've had a poor night of sleep, you can't change it. You now have absolutely no control over that poor night's sleep whatsoever.

But you can control how you think about it. You can change the meaning you give to it.

'Brilliant, I slept poorly, so I will use this day to help strengthen my sleep drive and condition my brain that a poor night of sleep is not a threat, so I sleep even better over the long run.'

Sounds fantastic!

And really, what's the alternative? Wishing you had slept better and doing everything you can to make yourself more miserable than when you first woke up. That doesn't sound great to me.

> 'You can't go back and make a new start, but you can start right now and make a brand new ending.' (Sherman, 1982)

> 'You're a wonderful human being. Please don't punish yourself for not sleeping by watching *Here Comes Honey Boo Boo*.' (Joseph Pannell, 2021)

25

Beyond CBT-I

I had finished my sleep course, and I was on my own now. Now comes the moment to continue my new behaviours and thought patterns so I could continue to sleep well.

This sounds like it could be difficult, but it wasn't. It was actually harder for me not to. During most of the course, I had used willpower to do the new habits and behaviours. Getting out of bed in the morning at more or less the same time every day was a challenge.

It got much easier as the course progressed, but it never came naturally. Because I saw results, I put the effort in, and the results kept coming. A week or two after finishing my course, things started to change.

A couple of weeks after my course ended, most mornings, I would wake before the alarm. The sluggishness and the force required to rise wasn't there anymore, and it just became automatic to get out of bed.

The willpower and effort had gone. Slowly but surely, through repetition and consistency (not perfection, just good enough), my new behaviours had started to become habits.

In fact, they weren't new behaviours anymore. They were just what I did. They were becoming part of my identity. I get up at the same time every day. That's just what I do!

And as the new behaviours became part of my identity so did the new thought patterns. The course had proved to me that I could sleep and that the less effort I put into sleeping in the short term, the more I slept over the long term. Less effort had now become as much of a habit and part of my identity as getting up at the same time every day. I don't force or try to sleep. That's just what I do!

I had achieved more than I could ever have hoped. Most nights, I was sleeping amazingly, spending the majority of my time in bed asleep and feeling incredible the next day.

I was no longer scared to go to bed anymore as I knew that when I did, I would sleep, and that if I didn't, it didn't matter. As long as I didn't try to change anything, I would sleep well the next night.

But there were still a couple of active sleep efforts that I struggled to let go of.

A month after finishing my sleep course, I was still restricting my time in bed to 7 hours. Two months after the course, I was still restricting my sleep to 7 hours.

A quarter of an hour at a time, I had built up to 7 hours, and then I stopped. I don't want any more time in bed, I told myself, so why would I want to stop restricting my time in bed?

I had been helped to come off my sleep window during the last session of my course, but after finishing my course, I still wanted to be on that sleep window, and I struggled to let it go.

Why?

Well, my sleep window gave me something concrete that I could cling to that I thought would make me sleep. It gave me certainty. I had spent twenty years looking for this certainty, and no matter how many hot baths and kiwi fruit I had, I had never found it. And now I had got it. Sleep windows were something that virtually guaranteed me healthy natural sleep.

Why would I want to let that go?

I was fearful. Sleep windows work. Incredibly well. What if I actively stop restricting my sleep and I go back to being an *insomniac*, I asked myself?

Before, I had put my confidence in my ability to sleep on supplements, kiwis etc. Now I had put my confidence in my ability to sleep to my sleep window.

My sleep window makes me sleep.

Does it? Or was I sleeping because I now had a regulated sleep drive and I was no longer hyperaroused.

If you are sleepy and you are not hyperaroused, you will sleep.

I had let go of all my other active sleep efforts and had slept wonderfully, so why not my sleep window too? What if there were a technique I could use to make doing so completely effortless? Well, luckily, there is!

Sleep Knowledge 25
The timeless night

The timeless night is a very effective way to transition off your sleep window. I learnt this technique from Michael Schwartz.

It works like this.

Now that you have a good idea of when you typically start to feel sleepy, set yourself a time after which you never look at a clock again.

In my example, my sleep window started at 11.30 pm and, because I now had a regulated sleep drive, I would generally start to feel sleepy as 11.30 pm approached.

I chose 10 pm for my timeless night to begin. After this time, I never looked at a clock again until my alarm sounded in the morning.

What this does is three things:

1) It stops you from setting your bedtime by your watch.

2) It prevents you from spending hours on your phone or laptop when you could be enjoying yourself and relaxing. (There are time displays on laptops and phones, so they're out!)

3) It stops you clock-watching and worrying and obsessing about the time when you are in bed.

Say you woke up in the middle of the night and then fell back asleep, usually, you would know almost exactly how long you were awake during the night because you looked at the time when you woke. Now you don't. Who knows what time you woke up and what time you fell back asleep, and who knows how many hours you slept last night? Sleep is a natural process, and your body will sleep when it needs to, so why does it matter how long you have slept?

Remember the buffer zone from an earlier Sleep Knowledge section? Now you can do both at the same time.

At 10.30 pm the buffer zone starts and, also at 10.30 pm, the timeless night starts: time for yourself to do the things you love before bed. (How much time after 10.30? You have no clock, so who knows!) No setting your bedtime by your watch and no obsessing about the time during the night. Good stuff!

Using the timeless night during your sleep window is incredibly helpful too. You won't be able to use it fully because you are sticking to a sleep window where you go to bed after a certain time, so you're going to need to know the time for that. But once your sleep window has begun, banish the clocks!

26

Improvements and Setbacks

The course was complete. On the day the course finished, had I ultimately resolved every one of my anxious thoughts around sleep, and could I truthfully say that I was now a normal sleeper? No.

I could, however, truthfully say that I was a good 80%–90% there, and I had absolute confidence that I would eventually get to a place where I could call myself a normal sleeper.

After my course ended, I did still very occasionally take sleeping tablets. Sleeping tablets were, for me, the thing that took a little more time to phase out slowly.

On reflection, I think this was because over the fifteen years or so of taking them, they were the thing that I had placed the most confidence in.

Nevertheless, from the moment the course finished, I can truthfully say that I was taking them much less frequently and that the dose I was taking was also considerably lower.

Before the course, I took a whole tablet. In the early stages, three-quarters. Towards the end, a half. As my confidence in my innate ability to sleep grew and grew after the end of the course within two months of completion, I was down to a third;

after three months, a quarter. Four months on, I took a razor blade to a tablet to shave off probably an eighth.

An eighth of a tablet was so small I couldn't even pick it up. It was when I caught myself pulling out a pair of tweezers that I pulled myself up short and laughed at myself.

'What on earth are you doing, Joseph?' I said. 'A door mouse could swallow a dose like that and run a mile.'

Throughout the time I had been taking these tiny doses, had I been sleeping all by myself? Of course, I had!

There and then I dumped the rest of the packet in the bin, and I have never taken them again.

Stopping sleeping pills entirely during the course would have been perfect.

Feeling confident enough to quit sleeping tablets five months after my course completion was good enough. And good enough, really is good enough.

Is that the end of the story? The day I dumped the sleeping pills in the bin, was I a normal sleeper? I would love to say yes, as I thought I was, but I wasn't. A couple of weeks later, I had a setback – a big one.

When you overcome insomnia, progress isn't linear. During the months following the course, my sleep got progressively better and better, but there were times when it didn't.

Sometimes my sleep was worse than the previous week, and I could pinpoint nothing to say why. It just was. But always without fail, as long as I stuck to my new behaviours and didn't go down the rabbit hole of forcing or protecting sleep, it would normalise again, and my sleep would get right back on track and continue to improve progressively.

Except when it didn't.

Break-up, business loss ... Things had taken a turn for the worse for me. But now everything seemed to be going my way, and life was getting better. Sometimes, however, when things are going well, the cosmos likes to have a giggle and dump a load of crap on your doorstep that you didn't order.

It does that from time to time to see whether you'll complain and wallow in it, or whether you'll take it around the back to dig into your garden and grow some beautiful flowers in it.

It was another very stressful time in my life, and for one, two, three, four nights, I didn't sleep.

So I made a few adjustments to my behaviours. Not many. Just a few. And a few more, and a few more. Three weeks later, I was back exactly where I had started: taking supplements to force sleep, waking late to 'catch up' on sleep when it was on offer, the hot baths, the kiwi fruit, everything.

And with the old behaviours came the old thought patterns and the endless scrolling through the internet to figure out why I wasn't sleeping.

I had slept amazingly for six months, but now that had all gone.

I had it. And in the space of three weeks, I had lost it. I was devastated.

Sleep Knowledge 26
The reticular activating system and setbacks

The reticular activating system: a bundle of nerves in our brain stem that filters out information and teaches it what to notice and focus on.

A swift demonstration of how it works is in the exercise below. Read Step 1 and then do the exercise before reading Step 2 or it won't work. (I know I tricked you earlier by asking you to turn your hair blue, but this exercise is different and worth doing.)

Step 1

As quickly as you can, for 15 seconds, look around you and find everything you can that is red. Look for red, look for red, under the table, on the walls, as quick as you can, look for red.

Step 2

If you have read this step before doing the exercise, perhaps go back to step 1 first. It only takes 15 seconds.

Step 3

If you have read this step before doing the exercise, perhaps go back to step 1 first. It only takes 15 seconds.

Step 4

Which is actually Step 2. Close your eyes and try to think of everything you saw that was black.

That's how the reticular activating system works.

Those past six months, I had slept better than I ever had, but I chose to laser my focus in on the past three weeks when I hadn't slept and completely filtered out everything else. I did this because my sleeplessness was happening **now**.

Your brain is a survival machine, and the threat was immediate. What happens if I go back to being an insomniac? What will happen if I don't sleep tonight? What will happen if ...

But why was I not sleeping?

Firstly, normal sleepers go through short-term sleep difficulties, especially during stressful events (Hurray, I must be a normal sleeper!)

Secondly, I changed my behaviours from my new ones (sleep!) to my old ones (no sleep!).

When my behaviours changed from my new behaviours to my old behaviours, walking arm and arm were my old thought patterns. (Why can't I sleep? What can I do to sleep? What can I do to prevent this ever happening again?)

When you hit a speed bump, what can you do, then?

Thankfully, I had the answer.

Journalling.

For six weeks after I had finished my sleep course, I had kept a journal about my sleep. I wrote down all my successes, not just the times I slept well, which were many.

'I woke at the same time today for the fifteenth time running and yet again slept AMAZING!'

I also noted my successes with my thought patterns, when, like a normal sleeper, I had a poor night sleep.

'Last night I slept a little poorly but I got up, I got active, had a fantastic day and kept on trucking.'

I only wrote in the journal for six weeks. As my sleep improved, I let go of this too, but I still kept hold of the journal.

During my setback, I dug the journal out and read through it. Doing so shifted my focus away from my inability to sleep and back to my ability to sleep. I could sleep. It was there in black and white!

My new behaviours were reinstated, and very quickly after my new behaviours were reinstated, my new thought patterns followed suit. It didn't take weeks like the first time around for my hyperarousal to vanish. This was because I had conditioned my brain to link my new behaviours with sleep, so as soon as I put my new behaviours back in place, my thought patterns changed from the old, to the new ones almost instantly.

27

That's a Wrap Folks

As I write this, it is roughly a year and a half from the ink drying on my divorce papers.

I would not have said this during it, but now that I am through it, I can say with all sincerity that I am happy for our time together, but I wouldn't change the outcome for anything in the world.

As for my sleep ...

I no longer force sleep. I am no longer scared to go to bed or be in it, and I am no longer concerned when I wake during the night (everybody does!). My sleep receives no attention. Good night's sleep, poor night's sleep, no worries, no problem. However much I sleep on any given night is good enough – I make no effort to sleep more or sleep better, zero, zip.

The only thing I do now is go to bed when I'm sleepy, get up at more or less the same time every day, get loads of light and erm ... well that's about it.

And now that I don't try to sleep, guess how well I am sleeping. Amazingly!

The energy I have is fantastic. The shadow I had over my life has lifted. I now love the days again, and I'm back doing all the hobbies that made me me.

Now I have overcome my own insomnia, I enjoy nothing more than helping others sleep; it gives me meaning. When I hear somebody tell me how much better they are now sleeping, nothing in the world makes me happier. And to top it all, although it is early days, I have met somebody wonderful!

I said, when my insomnia was at its worst, that I would swap the rest of my life to sleep well for the next ten. I meant it.

I said it as a vain plea chucked into the wind that I never thought could happen.

While it wasn't easy, and I have taken a few backwards steps along the way, I now do sleep well.

Not perfectly, and not every night. I can't sleep on a washing line, but overall, I can now truthfully say that I am a reasonably good sleeper. And to say that truthfully is testament to just how far I have come and the power of the sleep knowledge and techniques that I have learnt from everybody who has taught me and that I have now shared with you in this book.

For twenty years, I never met anybody who understood insomnia; I always felt alone with it and that there was nothing I could do to overcome it.

The purpose of my writing this book was to help you feel validated and give you the certainty that your insomnia can and will be overcome.

Your insomnia might present differently from what I had, but it is still insomnia, and the door out of it is the same one I walked through. I have included at the back of this book further resources to help you. No matter where you are based in the world and no matter what your budget, there will be something for you.

I can now call myself a good sleeper. You may think I am lucky, but I am not. The only difference between you and me is that a year and a half ago, I found the most effective evidence-based cure for insomnia there is, committed to it, and did it.

Soon you will be able to call yourself a good sleeper too. Sleep is wonderful. I highly recommend it!

Afterword

Thank you for reading my book! I hope it will be of value to you.

It was a tricky decision for me to write it as, having obsessing about insomnia for twenty years, after I overcame it, a huge part of me would have liked to never think about sleep again.

That said, I hate to think that there are so many millions of people with insomnia when I know that, with the right sleep knowledge, they don't have to have it, so now I'm determined to get this book to as many of them as possible.

Helping people sleep feels amazing. If this book has helped you and you would like to help someone you know sleep (or perhaps someone you don't know!), please consider leaving a review and/or sharing the 10 Gold-Standard Techniques to Overcome Insomnia **(see Appendix below) on your social media, blog or website.**

You can find them in an easily social-media-shareable copy-and-paste format and as a video on my website: www.youcansleeptoo.com, as well as on my Facebook page, which you can find by searching 'You Can Sleep Too!'

On my website, I also have a tonne of other resources and recommended YouTube videos to help you with your sleep, and I will be adding new content frequently.

Appendix

10 Gold-Standard Techniques to Overcome Insomnia

1) Only go to bed when you are can't-keep-your-eyes-open sleepy.

Sleep is a drive state. Just as you have a drive to eat when you feel hungry, you also have a drive to sleep when you feel sleepy.

It is a common belief that you should set a fixed bedtime. Setting your bedtime by your watch rather than based on how you feel causes you to spend more time in bed trying to force sleep and becoming anxious if it doesn't come. Go to bed when you physically can't keep your eyes open and sleep feels irresistible!

2) If you are in bed and feeling worried about not sleeping, leave the bedroom.

If you are in bed not asleep, think about how you feel. If you are sleepy, relaxed and just as happy to be in bed awake as you are asleep. Wonderful!

If you stay there, do nothing and allow sleep to come, it will.

If you start to feel anxious about not sleeping and are trying to force sleep, give yourself permission to leave the bedroom and do something you find relaxing and enjoyable. When you feel sleepy again, return to bed.

3) Get up at the same time every day.

Getting up at the same time every day is one of the most essential pieces of advice to improve your sleep because a regular wake time anchors your circadian rhythm and homoeostatic sleep drive.

Even when you sleep poorly, if you can resist the urge to sleep late so that you can catch up on sleep in the short term, you will see a dramatic improvement in your sleep over the long term.

4) Get light!

Get plenty of light (natural or artificial) as soon as possible and throughout the first third of your day.

5) Don't believe the 8-hour sleep myth.

Objectively measured in a sleep lab, most adults who do not have a sleep problem sleep between 5.5 and 7 hours and overestimate the amount of sleep they actually get by about an hour.

Some people may need 8 hours of sleep, but this is not typical. Everybody is different. The amount of sleep you personally need is enough for you to feel happy and refreshed. That's it!

6) Spend less time in bed.

People with insomnia typically try to force sleep by spending more time in bed. Doing so serves to increase the amount of time spent in bed awake in an anxious, hyperaroused state; this conditions the brain to see the bed as a place of worry and wakefulness rather than sleep.

The fastest way to regulate your sleep drive and tackle the hyperarousal that can mask your drive to sleep is to spend less time in bed.

7) Understand what causes and perpetuates insomnia.

Stressful events, ailments and medication can all cause a short-term sleep problem. Normal sleepers have short-term sleep problems too. What causes and allows insomnia to continue are behaviours to try to force and catch up on sleep (napping, sleeping late, going to bed early when you are not sleepy) and your anxiety around sleep (your hyperaroused state).

Insomnia **always** boils down to two problems: unregulated sleep drive and hyperarousal.

Your insomnia is not unique. Knowing this with absolute certainty gives you the confidence it can be resolved.

8) Be mindful of active sleep efforts.

Hot baths, kiwi fruit, meditation, supplements, sleeping on the left side of the bed, sleeping at the north end ... These are all active sleep efforts to try to force sleep. Just as it is impossible to turn your hair blue using breathing exercises, it is impossible to make yourself sleep if you are not already sleepy.

Hot baths and breathing excerises feel great, but if you have a laundry list of things you must do in order to sleep, this only increases your anxiety.

9) Be mindful of avoidance sleep efforts.

If I want to sleep, I can't go out with friends and drink **any** alcohol. I can't go out to a restaurant and eat late. I can't exercise after a certain time. I can't, I can't, I can't. All of these things mentioned may **have an** impact on sleep in the short term, but normal sleepers still do them and they still sleep.

Avoidance sleep efforts limit your life, lead to loss of control and agency over it, and increase the power that insomnia has over you. This **will** damage your sleep over the long term. **If it's 9 pm and you want to go roller skating, get stuck in!**

10) Get read up.

If these techniques have already been of value, imagine what an entire book will do for you. Grab yourself a copy of *You Can Sleep Too!* by Joseph Pannell. I had insomnia for two decades, and I put it to bed with the gold-standard, evidence-based treatment. So can you!

Resources

Daniel Erichsen and Michael Schwartz:
https://www.thesleepcoachschool.com/

My sleep tutors! Sleep physiologist Daniel Erichsen and sleep coach Michael Schwartz have a vast array of excellent videos on Youtube. They are kind, compassionate sleep specialists with decades of experience, incredible knowledge and a clear, accessible way of sharing it.

I quote Daniel's book *Set It & Forget It* because quite frankly it is brilliant! And I have it on good authority that Daniel has a new one coming out very shortly.

On his website, he also has an online sleep course, and you can find his sleep app at https://bedtyme.co/.

Stephanie Romiszewski: https://sleepyheadclinic.co.uk
https://sleepyheadprogram.com/

Possibly the most knowledgeable, experienced sleep physiologist on the entire planet, I first found Stephanie Romiszewski and Sleepyhead Clinic on YouTube and have since learnt a considerable amount from them, so I owe her a lot.

I would highly recommend the online video course. (Remember your insomnia is not unique, everybody's insomnia is the same, so this course will work for you!) It is available to purchase on the Sleepyhead Clinic website or at https://sleepyheadprogram.com/.

This is a step-by-step, week-by-week, sleep course that you can access at any time from anywhere in the world and that is yours to keep forever!

Sleepyhead clinic also has free advice on their Facebook page and some fantastic videos on You Tube. I would recommend: 'Sleeping the Night Away with Stephanie Romiszewski' and 'Stephanie Romiszewski | How to Achieve Deep, Restful Sleep'.

Martin Reed: https://insomniacoach.com/about/

Last, but certainly not least, I present to you the hugely talented and experienced Martin Reed.

You can find Martin Reed on his website, where you can purchase online or phone coaching. He also has a **free** (get in!) email course you can follow and a podcast page.

He also has hundreds of videos on YouTube which you can find by typing 'Martin Reed Insomnia'.

Incredibly accessible, easy-to-follow teaching presented in a clear and concise way. Martin is absolutely fantastic at what he does. I could not recommend him highly enough!

You can find all the books and articles that I quoted during my book in the References section that follows.

So, there we have it: online courses, free YouTube videos, a recommended book and an app. Sorted! I will post all these links and all the YouTube videos I recommend on my website http://www.youcansleeptoo.com/.

References

Blume, Christine, Corrado Garbazza and Manuel Spitschan (2019). 'Effects of Light on Circadian Ryhthm and Mood'. *Somnologie* 23(3): 147–156. https://www.ncbi.nlm.nih.gov/pmc/articles/PMC6751071/

Brahm, Ajahn (2015). 'Two Bad Bricks in the Wall' in *Opening the Door of Your Heart: And Other Buddhist Tales of Happiness*. Hachette Australia.

Division of Sleep Medicine at Harvard Medical School (2007). 'The Drive to Sleep and Our Internal Clock'. *Healthy Sleep*. http://healthysleep.med.harvard.edu/healthy/science/how/internal-clock

Erichsen, Daniel (2019). 'Don't worry about your health'. *BedTyme*. https://bedtyme.co/2019/12/06/3479/.

Erichsen, Daniel (2020). *Set It & Forget It: Are You Ready to Transform Your Sleep?* Independently published.

Harvey, Alison G. and Nicole K. Tang (2012). '(Mis)perception of Sleep in Insomnia: A Puzzle and a Resolution'. *Psychological Bulletin* 138(1): 77–101. https://www.ncbi.nlm.nih.gov/pmc/articles/PMC3277880/

Junger, Sebastian (2017). *Tribe: On Homecoming and Belonging*. Fourth Estate.

Lin, Hsiao-Han, Pei-Shan Tsai, Su-Chen Fang and Jen-Fang Liu. (2011). 'Effect of Kiwifruit Consumption on Sleep Quality in Adults with Sleep Problems'. *Asia Pacific Journal of Clinical Nutrition* 20(2): 169–174. https://pubmed.ncbi.nlm.nih.gov/21669584/

McLeod, Saul A. (2018). 'Classical Conditioning'. *Simply Psychology.* https://www.simplypsychology.org/classical-conditioning.html

Mitchell, Matthew D., Philip Gehrman, Michael Perlis and Craig A. Umscheid (2012). 'Comparative Effectiveness of Cognitive Behavioral Therapy for Insomnia: A Systematic Review'. *BMC Family Practice*13: 40. https://www.ncbi.nlm.nih.gov/pmc/articles/PMC3481424/

Murakami, Haruki (2002). *Dance, Dance, Dance.* **Vintage.**

Robbins, Anthony (2003 [1991]). *Awaken the Giant Within.* Simon and Schuster.

Romisewski, S, F.E.K May, E.J. Homan, B. Norris, M.A. Miller, A. Zeman (2020). 'Medical Student Education in Sleep and Its Disorders Is Still Meagre 20 Years On: A Cross-Sectional Survey of UK Undergraduate Medical Education'. *Journal of Sleep Research* 29(6):e12980. https://pubmed.ncbi.nlm.nih.gov/32166824/.

Sherman, James R. (1982). *Rejection: How to Survive Rejection and Promote Acceptance.* **Pathway Books.**

Thompson, Richard (1994). 'Beeswing' on *Mirror Blue.*
Capitol.

University of Manchester (2019). 'Blue Light May Not Be
as Disruptive to Our Sleep Patterns as Originally
Thought'. *ScienceDaily* 16 December 2019.
www.sciencedaily.com/releases/2019/12/191216173654.htm.

Printed in Great Britain
by Amazon